100 HEALTH-BOOSTING
FOODS

100 HEALTH-BOOSTING FOODS

facts and recipes for super health

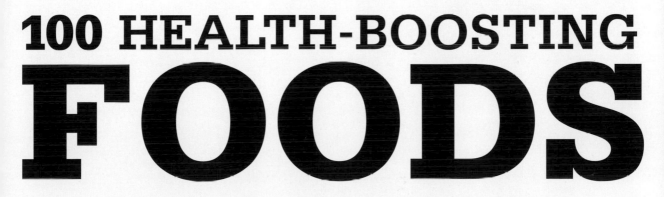

hamlyn

An Hachette UK company
www.hachette.co.uk

First published in Great Britain in 2007
by Hamlyn, a division of Octopus
Publishing Group Ltd
Endeavour House
189 Shaftesbury Avenue
London WC2H 8JY
www.octopusbooks.co.uk

This edition published in 2015

ISBN 978-0-600-63067-8

A CIP catalogue record for this book is
available from the British Library.

Printed and bound in China

10 9 8 7 6 5 4 3 2 1

Notes

Both metric and imperial measurements are given for the recipes.
Use one set of measures only, not a mixture of both.

Ovens should be preheated to the specified temperature. If using a
fan-assisted oven, follow the manufacturer's instructions for
adjusting the time and temperature. Grills should also be
preheated.

This books includes dishes made with nuts and nut derivatives. It
is advisable for those with known allergic reactions to nuts and nut
derivatives and those who may be potentially vulnerable to these
allergies, such as pregnant and nursing mothers, invalids, the
elderly, babies and children, to avoid dishes made with nuts and
nut oils. It is also prudent to check the labels of preprepared
ingredients for the possible inclusion of nut derivatives.

The Department of Health advises that eggs should not be
consumed raw. This book contains some dishes made with raw or
lightly cooked eggs. It is prudent for more vulnerable people such
as pregnant and nursing mothers, invalids, the elderly, babies and
young children to avoid uncooked or lightly cooked dishes made
with eggs.

Meat and poultry should be cooked thoroughly. To test if poultry is
cooked, pierce the flesh through the thickest part with a skewer or
fork – the juices should run clear, never pink or red.

Safety note

This book should not be considered a replacement for professional
medical treatment; a physician should be consulted on all matters
relating to health. While the advice and information in this book is
believed to be accurate, neither the author nor publisher can
accept any legal responsibility for any injury or illness
sustained while following it.

contents

introduction 6

eating your way to health 8

healthy eating 10

carbohydrates 14

proteins 16

fats 18

vitamins 20

minerals 22

phytonutrients 24

health-boosting foods at a glance 26

nutrients and phytonutrients 30

preserving nutrients 32

health conditions and complaints 34

the 100 foods 38

glossary 240

index 252

acknowledgements 256

introduction

The very fact that you're reading this book shows that you are interested in your health or that of your loved ones. It is certainly a subject that should concern all of us; time and again scientific research has linked diets rich in certain foods with better health and the absence of particular diseases. For example, the low incidence of serious disease among Mediterranean populations is attributed to specific foods in their diet (seafood, tomatoes, olive oil and red wine).

Since most of us choose what we eat we are, to some extent, responsible for our own health. We need a balanced diet that provides all of the necessary vitamins, minerals, protein, carbohydrates, fibre and fats to maintain our health and wellbeing. You may be tired of hearing the phrase 'we are what we eat' but it accurately reflects the fact that our food does more than just satisfy pangs of hunger. It helps the body grow, repair and regenerate cells; function efficiently and fight off infection. It therefore makes sense to choose the best foods possible for the purpose – foods that are rich in nutrients and have been linked with specific health benefits.

What are health-boosting foods?

Currently there is a great deal of interest in the health-boosting properties of certain foods, often referred to as 'superfoods' or 'miracle foods'. Ongoing research studies and scientific analysis have demonstrated the specific health benefits of certain foods. For example, cruciferous vegetables like broccoli and cabbage have been strongly linked with a decreased risk of cancer, while oily fish is believed to help protect against heart disease.

This book concentrates on 100 top foods that can help boost your health. These foods work in various ways depending on their specific composition of nutrients and phytonutrients (chemicals derived from plants). Many contain antioxidants, beneficial nutrients that help protect against infections and diseases and slow down the ageing processes in the body.

Besides promoting good general health, some of the health-boosting foods in this book are particularly important for tackling specific conditions, for example insomnia and high blood pressure. Some are very important for people who are stressed; others make you look better, improving the appearance of skin and complexion, and strengthening teeth and nails.

Boosting your wellbeing

You don't need to become obsessive about your health, but knowing which foods are health-boosters can help you make good choices. Doing the best you can for your health by regularly eating foods that provide good-quality fuel for your body has other benefits. It can make you feel good from within and more optimistic in general. It should also give you more energy, and take away the sluggishness caused by too much junk food.

eating your way to health

10

healthy eating

Experts believe that many of the ills suffered by modern industrialized western societies are largely due to diet and lack of regular physical activity. This book focuses on the nutrient-rich foods you should be eating but, on the subject of physical activity, most of us probably need to increase the amount we do. Simply walking more everyday, instead of using cars, escalators and lifts, is a good starting point. Beyond that, try and make exercise a routine part of life instead of an occasional extra.

Good nutrition

The importance of good nutrition – at all stages of our lives – cannot be overemphasized. It lies at the very heart of good health since the cells in our bodies, essentially the body's building blocks, rely on a good supply of nutrients in the diet to create and continually renew all the tissue and organs in the body. The *essential* nutrients required by our bodies are carbohydrates, protein, fats, vitamins and minerals (phytonutrients – see page 24 – are a bonus). Without the vital nutrients cellular health, and therefore general health, is adversely affected as cells that function inefficiently result in low energy levels, premature ageing and disease.

Variety

Apart from human milk, which alone provides for a baby's needs in the first few months of life, there is no one food that provides all the nutrients our bodies need. However nutrient-rich it may be, eating loads of just one type of food is rarely good for us. On the contrary, we need to eat a wide variety of foods, from all of the main food groups (see below), so as to benefit from all of the different nutrients available. In addition, different nutrients tend to interact and work in synergy. For example Vitamins C and E actually work together to make each other more effective – vitamin C recycles vitamin E, allowing it to carry on working longer.

Thinking ahead

What you eat has a huge impact on your health. It affects the way that you feel and look, how much energy you have and how healthy you are overall, not only now but longer term, too. A poor diet – and therefore poor cell function – will affect your future health. This aspect should not be ignored because, thanks largely to modern medicine and improvements in hygiene, most of us can expect to enjoy much longer life spans than earlier generations. Since we are likely to live longer let's enjoy those years in as good health as possible. We need to do all we possibly can to protect ourselves from the physical consequences of ageing. In practice this means looking at what we eat and drink and evaluating how our diets could be changed to meet our bodies' needs now and in the future.

A healthy balance

A healthy diet is primarily about balance. Our bodies need certain amounts of carbohydrates, proteins, fats, vitamins and minerals in order to function efficiently and, by eating sensibly, this can easily be achieved. With busy lifestyles and stressful jobs, it is all too easy to neglect our diets. But bear in mind that a balanced diet will boost health, energy and vitality and doesn't necessarily mean hours of preparation and cooking (see 'Shopping wisely', page 33).

The simplest way to ensure you are eating a nutritionally sound diet is to eat a wide variety of foods and to think of your food intake in terms of a plate containing foods from each of the five major food groups in varying proportions. Although many foods contain all the various different nutrients to some extent, some foods are predominantly carbohydrate, protein or fat, and are relatively easily recognized as such (see pages 14–19).

Bread, cereals and potatoes

This group of starchy carbohydrate foods is the major source of energy in the diet and should make up the biggest portion on your plate. The group includes wholegrain cereals, bread, pasta, rice, potatoes and yams. All the foods in this group are low in fat and high in starchy carbohydrates and dietary fibre.

Fruit and vegetables

These should make up the next biggest portion on your plate. Fruit and vegetables are low in fat, high in dietary fibre and rich in vitamins, minerals and other plant chemicals which are believed to play an important part in preventing many common illnesses such as heart disease, diabetes and cancer.

The food pyramid

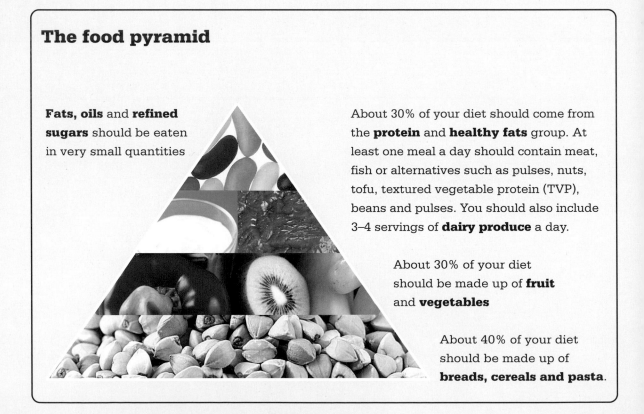

Fats, oils and **refined sugars** should be eaten in very small quantities

About 30% of your diet should come from the **protein** and **healthy fats** group. At least one meal a day should contain meat, fish or alternatives such as pulses, nuts, tofu, textured vegetable protein (TVP), beans and pulses. You should also include 3–4 servings of **dairy produce** a day.

About 30% of your diet should be made up of **fruit** and **vegetables**

About 40% of your diet should be made up of **breads, cereals and pasta**.

Dairy foods

Milk, cheese, yogurt and other dairy products should make up the third largest portion on your plate — choose low-fat dairy products to avoid too high an intake of fat. Milk and dairy foods supply our bodies with protein, calcium and zinc, and vitamins B_{12}, B_2, A and D.

Meat, fish and alternatives

Protein foods — lean meat, poultry, fish, lentils, pulses, eggs, soya products, nuts and seeds — should make up the fourth largest portion on your plate. Many of these foods are also good sources of B vitamins and minerals such as iron, calcium, magnesium and zinc.

Fats and sugars

Foods containing fats and/or refined carbohydrate such as sugar and honey should take up the least space on the plate. Such foods include margarine, butter, cooking oils, oil-based dressings, ice cream, pastries, biscuits, confectionery and soft drinks. Some fat is essential in the diet but too much can lead to heart disease and obesity. Sugars provide calories yet very few nutrients, and too much sugar can result in weight gain and tooth decay.

Top tips for healthy eating

Healthy eating does not mean cutting out treats completely, it simply means achieving the correct balance in your diet, being aware of the food that you eat and following a few simple guidelines:

- Eat a variety of foods
- Maintain a healthy weight
- Always refuse second helpings if you need to watch your weight
- Eat plenty of fruit and vegetables and foods rich in starch and fibre
- Choose foods that are low in fat
- Restrict your use of salt and sugar in cooking and at table
- Eat small meals and healthy snacks throughout the day (known as 'grazing'), rather than eating two or three large meals
- Eat only when you are hungry, rather than for the sake of it
- Never go food shopping when you are hungry
- Don't buy the foods you find hard to resist. That way there will be no temptation in the cupboards at home
- Drink alcohol only in moderation

14

carbohydrates

Carbohydrate foods provide the energy the body needs to function, both physically and mentally. There are two types of carbohydrate – sugars and starches, formerly known as 'simple' and 'complex' carbohydrates, respectively. Typical sources of carbohydrate are grains, legumes, vegetables and fruits.

Starches versus sugars

Starchy foods are much better energy providers than sugary ones. Starchy foods include grains and their products, such as bread, pasta and breakfast cereals, and starchy vegetables like potatoes. Simple sugars are those found naturally in milk, fruits and some vegetables. Refined white sugar contains calories yet no nutrients, and is therefore of no nutritious value at all.

Starchy carbohydrates with a high fibre content, for example legumes and unrefined wholegrain foods that have lost nothing during their processing, are particularly good for you because high-fibre carbohydrates are digested at a slower rate. As a result the blood sugar level in the body doesn't rise as quickly, whereas low-fibre carbohydrates are digested more quickly and consequently raise blood sugar rapidly. Rapid rises in blood sugar are undesirable since they cause the body to produce increased levels of insulin, the hormone that helps regulate blood sugar levels. Over time, this can result in health problems like diabetes.

The effect of different foods on blood-sugar levels is now better understood and common foods are ranked according to the glycaemic index (GI) where 0 is good and 100 (refined sugar) is bad.

The other major advantages of starchy foods is that their bulkiness gives a feeling of fullness when eaten (particularly useful for slimmers) and the slow release of their carbohydrate helps to sustain energy over a long period of time. For this reason sportspeople usually eat a very starchy meal some hours before competing as an effective way of storing energy for slow release during a long, gruelling running race or a rugby match, for example.

Which are starchy foods?

Starchy foods include all sorts of true grains (wheat, oats, rye, barley, millet, corn) and similar foods like buckwheat, quinoa and rice; products made from them such as bread, tortillas, pasta, noodles, couscous, cornmeal and breakfast cereals; plus the starchy vegetables such as potatoes, peas, yams and plantain.

Many of these foods, particularly the wholegrain cereals, are valuable sources of important vitamins and minerals and many of them also contribute to the protein content of the diet.

Fibre

Plenty of dietary fibre (also called roughage) in the diet is important for slowing the release of sugars into the bloodstream; it also keeps the bowel healthily active (see 'Grains and pulses', page 28).

The best sources are wholegrain cereal foods, such as wholemeal bread, wholewheat pasta and brown rice. Vegetables and legumes (chickpeas, beans and lentils) are very good sources of fibre, and seeds and fruit (especially pears, prunes, figs and raspberries) also make an important contribution.

How much?

Nutritionists recommend that a high percentage – 40–50 per cent – of our daily calorie intake should come from unrefined carbohydrates.

To increase your intake of high-fibre carbohydrates, replace white bread, white rice and sugary breakfast cereal with unrefined versions – wholemeal bread, brown rice, porridge oats, bran flakes and wholewheat pasta. In addition, snack on dried fruit and use legumes as a base for hearty soups and stews.

16

proteins

Proteins are the basic building blocks that are found in all cells in our bodies. They make up the structure of the cells as well as the elements inside, including enzymes and hormones. These structural elements are constantly being worn out so they need to be replaced by new proteins from our food.

What are proteins?

Proteins, found mainly in meat, fish, eggs, dairy products, grains, beans, peas, lentils and soya products are made up of chains of amino acids. There are about 20 different amino acids and the order in which they are linked in the chain depends on the type of protein they are making, be it a grain of wheat or muscle tissue in a cow. When we digest and absorb these foods, the chains are broken down into the individual amino acids. Our bodies then build up new chains with the amino acids in the right order to form different parts of the human body such as hair, muscle or a hormone.

Vegetable versus animal protein

It used to be thought that proteins from vegetable sources, such as grains and beans, were of a lower quality than those from animal sources such as meat and eggs, but it has since been shown that this is not true. They do have less protein per unit weight than meat products but the quality is the same. Overall, vegetable proteins such as bread, pasta, beans and lentils are a healthier option as vegetables and grains contain more fibre and a lot less fat than animal protein foods such as meat, cheese and milk.

Dairy products

Products such as milk, yogurt and cheese are good sources of protein and also provide essential minerals and vitamins. Milk is a very important source of calcium and also of the B vitamin, riboflavin. With the exception of children under two years who need whole milk for their development, most of us should use low-fat dairy products. Much of the content of fat-soluble vitamins (A, D, E) is lost, but the essential minerals such as calcium are still available.

Why do we need proteins?

Every cell in our bodies is partly composed of protein. We need adequate supplies of protein to build cells, and for the existing cells to go through their continuous process of growing and replacing themselves. We need to eat protein every day because our bodies can't store it – you cannot stock up on protein by eating large amounts of it once a week. As well as their role as building blocks, proteins, like carbohydrates, supply us with energy to fuel our bodies.

To compare, 1 g of protein supplies 4 calories, whereas 1 g of carbohydrate supplies 3.5 calories and 1 g of fat supplies 9 calories. If we are low on energy, our bodies will use proteins for fuel first but this is rather like fuelling a furnace with paper money since, unlike fats and carbohydrates, proteins have a much more important structural role, too.

The recommended protein intake in the diet is about 10 per cent of the total calories consumed.

18

fats

Our bodies need some fat for energy, internal processes and for the fat-soluble vitamins (vitamins A, D, E and K). The body can make all the fatty acids it requires except for the so-called essential fatty acids, which must be acquired from the diet. However, all fats are high in calories so it's advisable to restrict the total amount of fat in the diet to maintain a healthy weight as well as to control unhealthy blood cholesterol levels.

Cholesterol

This is a natural and necessary form of fat manufactured in the body from dietary fats. There are two types: 'good' cholesterol (high-density lipoprotein, HDL) and 'bad' cholesterol (low-density lipoprotein, LDL). Too much of the latter can clog the arteries, leading to heart disease and strokes. High levels of blood cholesterol may be reduced by restricting fat in the diet, especially saturated fat.

The different types of fat

The prime sources of fat in our diets are dairy products, meat, oils and fried foods. The main types of fat are saturated fats, trans fats, monounsaturated fats and polyunsaturated fats.

Saturated and trans fats

Usually solid at room temperature, saturated fats come mostly from animal sources – the fat on meat, butter, lard, cream and cheese – although vegetable sources include coconut butter and palm oil. A high concentration of saturated fat in the diet raises blood cholesterol levels, increasing the risk of blocked arteries, stroke and heart disease.

The process of hardening vegetable oil to make margarine is called hydrogenation and results in the production of trans fats. Trans fats are the worst fat of all for the heart and have been linked with an increased risk of breast cancer. They are also particularly harmful to diabetics as they interfere with insulin receptors responsible for control of blood sugar.

High quantities of saturated fats and trans fats are found in many fast foods as well as in processed foods such as biscuits, cakes and pastries.

Eating less fat

- **Choose lower-fat versions of dairy products, e.g. skimmed and semi-skimmed milk and reduced-fat cheese**
- **Use less fat in cooking. Grill and bake instead of frying and roasting**
- **Opt for low-fat spreads**
- **Use lean cuts of meat and remove the skin from poultry.**

Monounsaturated fats

Olive oil, rapeseed oil, avocados and many nuts are sources of monounsaturated fat. These fats help maintain healthy cholesterol levels and are thought to protect against heart disease.

Polyunsaturated fats

These fats include the essential fatty acids (omega-3 and omega-6 fats) our bodies require from our diet, and which help decrease the harmful LDL cholesterol level in blood. Good sources are fresh nuts and seeds and their oils (such as sunflower and walnut oils), leafy green vegetables, seafood and oily fish. Essential fatty acids should account for at least 15 per cent of our calorie intake. Most people get plenty of omega-6 fats in their diet (due to the widespread use of polyunsaturated oils) but need to focus on consuming more omega-3s.

Everyday fats

Butter and margarine have the same calorie content, whether or not the margarine is marked 'polyunsaturated'. Butter is a good source of the fat-soluble vitamins A and D, which are added to margarine. Low-fat spreads have a high water content and therefore a lower calorie content than butter or margarine. Most low-fat spreads have added fat-soluble vitamins.

Most cheeses have a high fat content. Quark is very low in fat, as are low-fat ricotta and fromage frais. Double cream is 50 per cent fat.

vitamins

There are two main types of vitamins – fat-soluble and water-soluble ones. The fat-soluble vitamins, A, D, E and K, are stored in the body and taking excessive amounts of them could be harmful. The water-soluble vitamins, vitamin C and the B complex vitamins, are not stored in the body and are therefore needed in the diet everyday. Any excess amounts of these are excreted in the urine.

Vitamin A and beta-carotene

An antioxidant, vitamin A is essential for vision in dim light and for the maintenance of healthy skin and surface tissues. It is stored in the liver and is toxic in excessive amounts. Vitamin A is found in cheese, eggs, whole milk and butter, and liver has a very high content.

Vitamin A can also be made in the body from beta-carotene (often referred to as its precursor), which is found in leafy green vegetables and in orange-coloured fruit and vegetables such as carrots and apricots.

Vitamin D

Vitamin D is essential for maintaining healthy levels of calcium and phosphorus in the body and for building healthy bones and teeth.

Deficiency causes rickets in children and osteomalacia (bone thinning) in adults.

The body makes its own vitamin D through the action of sunlight on the skin. Dietary sources are of less importance, except for people who cannot go out or who do not expose their skin to the light. Sources include oily fish, milk, butter and egg yolks. Vitamin D is added to margarine, and some breakfast cereals and yogurts.

Vitamin E

One of the top antioxidants, Vitamin E fights free radicals (see page 24) and helps skin stay healthy. It is found in poultry, fish, vegetables, vegetable oils, wheatgerm, nuts and seeds.

Vitamin K

Vitamin K helps the body to make a number of proteins, one of which is necessary for blood clotting. It also helps prevent osteoporosis. It is found in leafy green vegetables, soya oil and margarine.

The B vitamins

The vitamin B complex comprises eight vitamins: thiamin (B1), riboflavin (B2), niacin (B3), pantothenic acid (B5), pyridoxine (B6), cobalamine (B12), biotin and folate (also known as folic acid).

Some of the B vitamins are essential for the release of energy from the food we eat; others are involved in making cells — some make nerve cells, which is why a deficiency of certain B vitamins may result in depression. B6, B12 and folate make red blood cells. These three also help protect the heart via their action on homocysteine while folate helps protect unborn babies against spina bifida.

The B vitamins are widely distributed in foods, including meat, milk, offal, fish, eggs, vegetables, fruit and wholegrains. Many breakfast cereals are fortified with B vitamins.

Vitamin C

Another antioxidant, vitamin C is needed for the growth and maintenance of healthy connective tissue, for boosting immunity and for helping the body absorb iron.

For humans, vitamin C must come from the diet. The best sources are certain fruits, particularly blackcurrants, strawberries, kiwi fruit, guavas and citrus fruits. Green salads and vegetables are also useful, particularly potatoes because of the large quantities generally eaten.

Vitamin C in fruits and vegetables diminishes with storing and cooking. Frozen vegetables may therefore sometimes have a higher vitamin C content than fresh vegetables that have been stored for some time.

Vitamin and mineral requirements

The amount of each vitamin and mineral we need changes according to our age, health, gender and level of activity.

- **Children generally need more vitamins as they are growing and active**
- **Pregnant women are advised to take supplements of folic acid in the first twelve weeks of pregnancy**
- **People over the age of 50 generally become less active so need less energy. It is therefore important that the food that they eat is more nutrient-dense than the average diet.**

minerals

Our bodies need minerals in the diet for the growth and maintenance of bones, cells and tissues. Some minerals, for example zinc, iron and chromium are needed in only very small quantities and are called trace minerals; others are required in much larger amounts. The more important dietary minerals are calcium, iron and zinc. Phosphorus and magnesium are also important, but a diet that provides sufficient calcium will also provide adequate phosphorus and magnesium.

Calcium

People of all ages, not just children, need calcium as it is vital for forming and continually strengthening bones and teeth. Calcium and phosphorus together form the framework of the skeleton. A deficiency of calcium may result in osteoporosis in later life, where calcium is lost from the bone, making it painful to bear weight. To prevent osteoporosis it is important to build strong bones early in life, when the bones are growing actively, through weight-bearing exercise and adequate dietary calcium.

Probably the most widely available sources of dietary calcium are milk, cheese and yogurt. Because the calcium in milk is in the watery part of the liquids, using skimmed or semi-skimmed milk, or low-fat yogurts and cheeses does not reduce calcium intake. Butter and cream contain very little calcium. Calcium is also naturally available in other foods, for example kale, tinned sardines, almonds and sesame seeds, and is often added to white bread, soya milk and tofu.

In addition to strengthening bones and teeth, calcium acts as a natural tranquillizer, soothing irritability and aiding insomnia.

Other dietary minerals

- Chromium (trace mineral): Works with insulin to balance blood sugar levels, helps lower cholesterol levels and protect against heart disease
- Copper (trace mineral): Helps the body use iron and convert food to energy
- Fluoride (trace mineral): Helps protect teeth
- Iodine (trace mineral): Helps control metabolic activity
- Magnesium: Helps cells and muscles work efficiently. Helps the body use calcium and potassium
- Manganese (trace mineral): An antioxidant and important for bone structure and nerve function

- Phosphorus: Required for healthy cells, bones and teeth
- Potassium: Helps in cellular growth and controlling blood pressure. Also good for the nervous system and for regulating bodily fluids and the acid—alkali balance in the body. Required for muscle activity and helps prevent cramp
- Selenium (trace mineral): A major antioxidant (see page 24) with anti-cancer powers
- Sodium: Helps regulate the body's water content and enables the nerves to function effectively.

Iron

Iron is particularly important for the formation of haemoglobin, the red pigment in blood. In theory we are born with enough iron to last through life, but if enough dietary iron is not eaten to restore any losses, anaemia can result.

The best sources of iron in the diet are red meat and liver because this iron is most easily absorbed. The iron in eggs is also well absorbed but the iron in vegetables or added to flour is less well absorbed. Consuming a source of vitamin C, such as orange juice or salad, with an iron-rich food helps the body absorb the iron. Tea inhibits absorption of iron, so avoid it around meal times.

Zinc

An antioxidant (see page 24), zinc is a trace mineral that helps in the healing of wounds, is involved in enzyme activity and is essential for healthy sex organs and male reproduction. It is present in a variety of foods – meat and dairy foods are good sources, as are nuts, wholegrains and seeds.

phytonutrients

Phytonutrients, which are also known as phytochemicals, are naturally occurring chemicals derived from plants. Unlike true nutrients (see pages 14–23), phytonutrients are not necessary for sustaining life but they are believed to actively help prevent ill health or diseases. They are particularly associated with preventing and/or treating cancer, heart disease, diabetes and high blood pressure.

Antioxidants

Antioxidants are powerful protective chemical compounds, which slow the rate of damaging oxidation in the body caused by free radicals. Free radicals are unstable oxygen molecules in our bodies generated by pollution, sunlight, cigarettes, certain foods, stress and normal metabolic processes such as breathing. Free radicals destabilize other, healthy molecules, initiating a chain reaction of cellular destruction and DNA degradation, resulting in accelerated ageing and degenerative conditions and diseases such as cataracts, atherosclerosis and cancer.

Uncooked fresh fruit and vegetables and most pulses are the best sources for antioxidants. Others include tea, red wine, olive oil, dark chocolate and many grains.

Useful phytonutrients

Flavonoids such as quercetin and ellagic acid and resveratrol (found in grapes and wine). Usually antioxidant, sometimes anti-inflammatory, sometimes antibiotic, flavonoids also have potent anti-carcinogenic properties. Some work by preventing cancer-promoting oestrogen from getting into cells, others suppress COX-2 (cyclo-oxygenase), an enzyme that enables cancer to grow and spread.

Anthocyanidins a class of flavonoids with very powerful antioxidant properties and thought to be 50 times more powerful than vitamin E. Abundant in red, purple and blue fruits, especially berries.

Carotenoids such as alpha-carotene, beta-carotene, lycopene, lutein, zeaxanthin. Powerful antioxidants with anti-cancer and anti-ageing properties.

Glucosinolates such as isothiocyanates, sulphoraphane, indoles. Anti-cancer compounds found in cruciferous vegetables.

How do antioxidants help us?

Eating antioxidant-rich foods helps prevent ill health as the antioxidants disarm the unstable molecules – slowing down, preventing or even reversing diseases resulting from cellular damage. Cancer cells, for example, are essentially normal cells that contain DNA damaged by free radicals. Because antioxidants stop free radicals and reduce DNA damage, they are a major defence against cancer.

As well as protecting us against serious degenerative diseases, antioxidants also boost the immune system, help prevent minor infections, reduce inflammation and help protect against conditions associated with premature ageing like skin wrinkling and memory loss.

Variety offers protection

There are over 4,000 different antioxidants – the key ones are vitamins A, C and E. The minerals selenium, manganese and zinc, some of the B vitamins and certain enzymes and amino acids also have antioxidant properties. Some antioxidants operate in water-soluble parts of the body, while others work in the fatty areas of cells and tissues. Some are better at fighting certain free radicals than others. A varied diet containing plenty of different antioxidant foods is therefore the best way to boost health, and why we should eat at least five portions of fruit and vegetables every day.

Top-scoring antioxidant foods

Using test-tube analysis, researchers from the Human Nutrition Research Center on Aging, Tufts University, Boston, US have rated foods according to their ability to quench damaging oxygen-free radicals, known as Oxygen Radical Absorbance Capacity. ORAC values are given as units per 100 grams (3½ oz) food.

Food	ORAC
Prunes	5770
Pomegranate	3037
Raisins	2830
Blueberries	2400
Blackberries	2036
Garlic	1940
Kale	1770
Strawberries	1540
Spinach	1260
Raspberries	1220
Brussels sprouts	980
Plums	949
Alfalfa sprouts	930
Broccoli florets	890
Beetroot	840
Oranges	750
Red grapes	739
Red pepper	710
Cherries	670
Kiwi fruit	602

26

health-boosting foods at a glance

Now that you know about all the different nutrients your body needs and how phytonutrients can boost health, you can start discovering which foods are the most nutritious. Health-boosting foods possess a high level of nutrients compared with their number of calories. The following pages list the top health-boosting foods – try and include them in your diet on a regular basis so as to reap the health benefits associated with eating them.

Fruit and vegetables

Numerous research studies have linked diets high in fruit and vegetables with less heart disease, cancer, high blood pressure and diabetes. Eat *at least* five portions (about 500 g/1 lb) per day, preferably more, of fruit and vegetables (excluding potatoes), especially the colourful fruit and vegetables as these are particularly rich in antioxidants and anti-cancer flavonoids and carotenoids. Research has shown that people who consume plenty of dark green, yellow, bright orange, deep red and purple produce have a significantly decreased risk of various cancers.

Fruit and vegetables — top health-boosters

açaí berries • alfalfa sprouts • apricots • asparagus • aubergines • avocados • bananas • beetroot (red beet) • berries • broccoli • brussels sprouts • butternut squash • cauliflower • cherries • chillies • corn on the cob • dates • fennel • figs • fresh herbs • garlic • ginger • globe artichokes • grapes • green beans • guavas • kale • kiwi fruit • mangetouts • mangoes • mushrooms • okra • olives • oranges • papayas • peas • peppers • pineapples • plums • pomegranates • potatoes • pumpkins • radishes • raisins • rhubarb • seaweed • spinach • swede • sweet potatoes • tomatoes • watercress • watermelons • yams

The high content of fibre in fruit and vegetables also has a big role in maintaining good health. A low-fibre diet causes constipation and over a period of time the bowel can lose its natural strength and elasticity. If there is too little fibre in the diet, the transit time of food residue is slowed, resulting in possible damage such as diverticulosis — the formation of small pockets in the lining of the gut. Too little fibre may also be a factor in the development of some forms of cancer. In addition, fibre helps to keep levels of blood cholesterol down and helps keep blood sugar levels steady.

Fish, meat and poultry

Everyone should eat at least two portions of fish per week to boost health, one of which should be oily. Fish is an excellent source of protein, vitamins and minerals, and is low in saturated fat. Oily fish (anchovies, herring, kippers, mackerel, salmon, sardines, tuna and whitebait) is particularly good because of its omega-3 fats, which are believed to help protect against heart disease, arthritis, breast cancer and dementia. (Because of the potential health risks from the levels of mercury in oily fish, women who are pregnant, breastfeeding or likely to have children in the future should eat no more than two portions per

Fish, meat and poultry — top health-boosters

anchovies • chicken • cod • game • guinea fowl • herrings • kippers • lean red meat • liver • mackerel • mussels • oysters • partridge • pheasant • prawns (shrimp) • salmon • sardines • scallops • snapper • tuna • turkey • venison • whitebait

27

Grains and pulses – top health-boosters

aduki beans • barley • black beans • borlotti beans • brown rice • buckwheat • butter beans • chickpeas • flageolet beans • kidney beans • lentils • millet • haricot beans • oats • pinto beans • quinoa • rye • soya beans • spelt • wheatgerm • wheatgrass and wheatgrass juice • wholegrain bread • wholewheat pasta

week; everyone else can eat up to four.)

Research suggests an association between red meat consumption and heart attack, stroke and bowel cancer. Certainly you should only ever eat lean red meat, and avoid meat products like sausages, burgers, black pudding, luncheon meat and salami.

Grains and pulses

People whose diets are rich in wholegrains and pulses tend to experience less stroke, heart disease, diabetes and cancer. Wholegrains and pulses lower cholesterol levels, which helps keep the heart healthy. They also maintain the health of the digestive and immune systems. By boosting fibre intake, wholegrains and pulses promote regular bowel movements which can help control some types of irritable bowel syndrome, avoid haemorrhoids (piles) and keep the intestines free of diseases such as diverticular disease and bowel cancer.

Wholegrains in the diet also improve blood sugar control, which helps prevent diabetes. In addition, they are rich in vitamin E, selenium and lignans, a type of phytoestrogen, all of which are associated with reduced risk of cancer. Compared with people who don't include wholegrains in their diet, those who eat wholemeal bread and pasta have been shown by a number of different scientific studies to have a 33 per cent lower risk of cancer and heart disease. Try and eat two to three portions of wholegrains every day.

Nuts and seeds

Regular consumers of nuts have been shown to have less risk of heart disease and diabetes than those who don't eat nuts.

Seeds contain all the essential nutrients for the growth of healthy new plants and are therefore often referred to as little

Nuts and seeds — top health-boosters

almonds • brazil nuts • cashews • hazelnuts • peanuts • pine nuts • walnuts • flaxseed (linseed) • poppy seeds • pumpkin seeds • sesame seeds • sunflower seeds

Other top health-boosters

Dark chocolate Raw cacao beans are rich in antioxidant flavonoids, so dark chocolate with the minimum of added milk and sugar may be considered a health-booster for its antioxidant powers. Cacao beans also contain high levels of some 'feel-good' neurotransmitters (serotonin, phenylethylamine and dopamine). Use real chocolate chips (crushed cacao beans) in cooking to benefit from this health-boosting food.
Spirulina A blue-green algae, spirulina is packed with natural goodness. It has antibacterial and antifungal properties and is good for anti-ageing. Use it in smoothies in its powdered form.

Other health-boosting foods include: reduced-fat **milk**, low-fat **live yogurt** and **cheese**, and **tofu**, all of which are high-calcium foods and therefore help prevent osteoporosis; **eggs**, **honey** and **molasses**, **olive oil** and tea.

'powerhouses of nutrition'. Try eating them as a snack or adding them to breakfast cereals, salads and stir-fries or to bread, biscuit and cake mixtures to boost energy levels and protect yourself against high cholesterol, anaemia, osteoporosis and heart disease.

30

nutrients & phytonutrients

Opinion is divided as to whether dietary supplements are necessary if you enjoy a balanced diet and eat a wide variety of health-boosting foods. Taking a daily multi-vitamin and mineral supplement may be a wise insurance policy for good health and certainly won't do you any harm. Bear in mind, however, that even the best one can't possibly replicate all the hundreds of vitamins, minerals and phytonutrients found in real foods.

Anthocyanidins Berries, cherries, red grapes

Beta-carotene Leafy green vegetables, carrots, pumpkin, butternut squash, apricots, canteloupe melons, mangoes

Biotin Chicken liver, kidney, meat, milk, eggs, beans, wholegrains, peanuts, almonds, sesame seeds

Calcium Tinned sardines, milk, cheese, yogurt, oats, beans, lentils, soya, tofu, beetroot, seaweed, spinach, kale, figs, almonds, cashews, walnuts, pumpkin and sesame seeds

Chromium Beef, chicken, shellfish, eggs, brown rice, wholemeal bread, brewer's yeast, peppers, nuts

Copper Fish, prawns, lamb's liver, tofu, seaweed, green vegetables, peanuts, cashew nuts

Folate (folic acid) Calf's liver, beans, lentils, fortified breakfast cereals, parsley, leafy green vegetables, spinach, romaine lettuce, watercress, broccoli, brussels sprouts, beetroot, asparagus, sweet potatoes, peanuts, sesame seeds

Fluoride Fish, tea

Iodine Fish, seafood, milk, eggs, seaweed, watercress, pears

Iron Red meat, liver, eggs, beans, lentils, soya, beetroot, broccoli, seaweed, sweet potatoes, watercress,

mangoes, papayas, pumpkin and sesame seeds

Isoflavones Soya beans and soya products

Lignans Rye, flaxseed (linseed)

Lycopene Tomatoes and processed tomato products, watermelon, guavas, pink grapefruit, rosehip

Manganese Egg yolks, beans, lentils, wholemeal bread, leafy green vegetables, okra, beetroot, tea, pineapple, blackberries, hazelnuts

Magnesium Prawns, wholegrains, beans, lentils, peas, soya, leafy green vegetables, peppers, sweet potatoes, beetroot, okra, pears, apples, berries, nuts, almonds, cashews, pumpkin and sesame seeds

Omega-3 essential fatty acids Oily fish, flaxseed (linseed), walnuts, mustard seeds

Omega-6 essential fatty acids Nuts and seeds

Phosphorus Fish, prawns, mussels, meat, turkey, dairy foods, eggs, sweet potatoes, apples, pears

Potassium Chicken, baked potatoes, bananas, prunes, dried apricots, almonds, peanuts

Selenium Prawns, salmon, snapper, meat, calf's liver, cheese, eggs, cereals, beans, lentils, soya, mushrooms, brazil nuts, walnuts, sesame seeds

Silicon Seaweed

Sodium Most raw foods contain small amounts of sodium chloride (salt) and it is widely found in ready meals and processed foods like crisps, bacon. We all consume too much salt and should halve our intake for the sake of our blood pressure

Sulphoraphane Cabbage, cauliflower, broccoli, kale, horseradish

Vitamin A (retinol) Oily fish, offal, whole milk, butter, cheese, eggs, beetroot, broccoli, cabbage, carrots, peppers, spinach, sweet potatoes, tomatoes, watercress, apples, pears, papayas, bananas, berries, cashews, chestnuts, hazelnuts, sunflower seeds

Vitamin B1 (thiamin) Cod's roe (taramasalata), game, wheatgerm, wholemeal bread, oatmeal, soya, peas, brazil nuts, peanuts

Vitamin B2 (riboflavin) Game, milk, yogurt, cheese, eggs, wheatgerm, broccoli, almonds

Vitamin B3 (niacin) Lamb's liver, tuna, salmon, sardines, halibut, venison, chicken, boiled eggs, wholemeal bread, soya, mushrooms, asparagus, peanuts

Vitamin B5 (pantothenic acid) Fish, meat (especially offal), egg yolks, beans, tofu, brewer's yeast, avocados, broccoli, peanuts

Vitamin B6 (pyridoxine) Fish, meat, eggs, wholegrains, soya, peppers, spinach, beetroot, bananas, hazelnuts

Vitamin B12 (cobalamine) Snapper, plaice, liver, milk, cheese, eggs, yeast extract, fortified breakfast cereals

Vitamin C (ascorbic acid) Potatoes, cauliflower, broccoli, kale, brussels sprouts, peppers, chillies, parsley, tomatoes, blackcurrants, strawberries, oranges, lemon juice, papayas, mangoes, guavas, kiwi fruit, brazil nuts, chestnuts, hazelnuts

Vitamin D (calciferol) Oily fish, cod liver oil, milk, butter, cheese, egg yolks, fotified margarine, fortified breakfast cereals, sunflower seeds

Vitamin E (tocopherol) Wheatgerm and wheatgerm oil, olive oil, soya oil, raw and dry-roasted nuts, sunflower and sesame seeds

Vitamin K Fish liver oil, liver, beans, peas, soya oil, margarine, potatoes, carrots, broccoli, brussels sprouts, spinach, leafy green vegetables, sunflower seeds

Zinc Sardines, oysters, crab, beef, lamb, calf's liver, game, cheese, eggs, soya, tofu, seaweed, tomatoes, hazelnuts, pine nuts, pumpkin and sesame seeds

preserving nutrients

Overreliance on processed convenience foods and drinks with all their chemical additives, extra salt, fat and sugar is undoubtedly a contributory factor to ill health in many Western societies today. Many of us are unfit and overweight and, as our bodies struggle to cope with the overload of toxins, we are more likely to succumb to infection and diseases. According to the World Health Organization dietary factors account for about 30 per cent of all cancers in the West.

Processed food

Processing food takes it a long way from its original state as a fresh whole ingredient packed with natural nutrients. For example polishing wholegrain rice to make white rice loses energizing B vitamins. Generally, the more a food is processed, the less nutrients remain. The exception to this is the lycopene in tomatoes. Because lycopene is fat soluble and tightly bound to fibre, crushing and/or cooking tomatoes makes the lycopene in products like canned tomatoes, tomato purée, tomato ketchup, tomato juice, spaghetti sauce and pizza, more easily absorbed by our bodies than that from raw tomatoes.

Healthy cooking and preparing

Cooking also destroys some nutrients which is why some people advocate a diet of totally raw whole foods and juices. Certainly, overcooking foods – for too long or at too high a temperature – can destroy many of their beneficial vitamins, minerals and phytonutrients, and may produce harmful free radicals (see page 24).

As a general rule, cook fruits and vegetables for as short a time as possible – steaming, microwaving or stir-frying are all good options if cooking is necessary. When boiling vegetables, add them to water that is already at a fast boil to shorten the cooking time and don't salt the water as this draws nutrients such as folate, potassium and vitamin C out of the vegetables where it is lost – unless you use the cooking water for making stock, sauces or gravy.

Avoid peeling fruit and vegetables so that you retain the minerals and vitamins which are frequently located just beneath the surface of the skin. To minimize nutrient loss prepare them only just before cooking to delay exposure to the air (oxidation), and never soak them in water.

Shopping wisely

All foods lose nutrients over time so shopping little and often ensures you always have fresh ingredients to hand – the fresher the food, the more nutrients it contains.

Rather than buying processed ready meals for an instant meal, choose natural convenience foods that cook speedily or require no cooking at all. You can quickly create delicious meals using salad ingredients; wholemeal breads like pitta; quick-cooking grains like couscous; pesto for instant pasta sauces; fresh herbs; tinned fish; grilled or griddled fresh meat or fish such as tuna, salmon or turkey steaks; baby new potatoes and steamed or microwaved fresh vegetables.

Buy only seasonal produce

Buying produce local to your area and in season ensures that it is very fresh, and therefore more nutritious than something picked while underripe, transported from the other side of the world, and ripened artificially in transit. In addition, seasonal produce is inevitably cheaper than imported foods.

Buy organic

Organic produce may be misshapen and covered with mud, but it often has more flavour than conventionally produced items where the emphasis is on appearance and long shelf life, often at the expense of nutrients. In addition, organic produce and organically farmed meat and poultry won't

have come into contact with chemicals that require your body to work harder to expel the toxins.

Correct storage

Storing food correctly is essential for preserving nutrients for as long as possible. Many ingredients, especially once cut open/started, need refrigerating to minimize further nutrient loss. Appropriate storage advice has been supplied for most of the 100 health-boosting foods in this book.

34

health conditions and complaints – what to eat

Including specific health-boosting foods regularly in your diet may help prevent or reduce the severity of the various conditions and diseases listed below. Use the information given here as a starting point but always consult your doctor for detailed medical and nutritional advice.

Anaemia
Eating iron-rich foods can help combat anaemia. Accompanying them with a vitamin C-rich food/drink will aid the body's absorption of the iron.

Eat more shellfish, red meat, offal, chicken, lentils, peas, green beans, dark green leafy vegetables (spinach, kale, watercress), dates, nuts

Drink less tea and coffee with meals as they inhibit iron absorption

Atherosclerosis
Atherosclerosis, a build-up of fatty deposits on artery walls, is a risk factor for heart disease, heart attack and stroke.

Eat more oily fish, wholegrains (especially oats), beans, lentils, soya, alliums (garlic, onions), tomatoes, olive oil, tea, cranberries, grapefruit, kiwi fruit, nuts (walnuts, almonds), seeds (sesame, pumpkin, sunflower)

Eat less saturated fats

Cellulite
Your diet can make a difference to the amount of cellulite you have.

Eat more beans, lentils, fibrous vegetables, apples and seeds to help eliminate waste and toxins and drink more water

Eat less refined and high-fat foods, salt, sugar, coffee and drink less tea and alcohol

Colds
You can't cure colds through diet but you can boost your immunity and alleviate the symptoms of a cold.

Eat more vitamin C-rich foods (citrus fruits, berries, kiwi fruit, green leafy vegetables), antibacterial foods (onions, garlic) and foods containing zinc to shorten the duration of colds (chickpeas, spinach, pumpkin seeds)

Eat less caffeine, dairy products (opinion is divided as to whether dairy foods encourage the production of mucus)

Constipation

Constipation is caused by a lack of fibre in the diet and is a risk factor for haemorrhoids, diverticulitis and bowel cancer. Make any dietary changes gradually to allow your digestive system to adapt.

Eat more insoluble fibre-rich foods (wholegrains, brown rice, wholemeal bread) and foods high in soluble fibre (porridge, beans, green leafy vegetables, apples, pears, apricots, figs, prunes), plus plenty of water

Eat less refined and processed foods

Depression

Focus on foods that boost your levels of the 'happy' brain chemical serotonin.

Eat more foods containing tryptophan (bread, potatoes, cauliflowers, bananas, dates, hazelnuts) and B vitamins (meat, offal, chicken, wholegrains, wheatgerm, pulses, most vegetables, yeast, nuts and seeds)

Drink less alcohol and caffeinated drinks

Exhaustion and fatigue

A better diet will keep you energized throughout the day.

Eat more oily fish, onions, garlic, nuts and seeds, low-glycaemic index carbohydrates (such as slow-release energy foods like oats), iron-rich foods (lean red meat, liver, spinach, apricots) and drink more water

Eat less: caffeine, saturated and trans fats, and high-glycaemic index carbohydrate foods e.g. cakes, pastries, soft drinks

Gout

You may be able to control gout (an excess of uric acid in the blood) with diet rather than medication.

Eat more lentils, green leafy vegetables, watercress, celery, beetroot, grapefruit, pineapple, cherries

Eat less protein-rich foods (fish, shellfish, red meat, offal, oats, mushrooms); fried foods and refined carbohydrates; very sweet fruit (such as grapes); sugar; drink less alcohol and coffee

Hangover

Speedy recovery involves drinking plenty of fluids and eliminating toxins from your system.

Eat more globe artichokes (to restore the liver); onions, garlic, green vegetables, apples, pears and citrus fruit (to help the body detoxify); low glycaemic index foods like porridge (to control your blood sugar levels). Drink more water and vitamin C-rich fruit juices (to rehydrate you)

Eat less saturated fats, processed foods; drink less coffee

High blood pressure (hypertension)

It is essential to reduce high blood pressure as it is a risk factor for stroke, heart disease and kidney disease.

Eat more: oily fish, high-fibre foods (oats, wholegrains, beans), soya, olive oil, alliums (garlic, onions, leeks, chives, spring onions), green leafy vegetables, broccoli, potatoes, beans, oats, celery, avocadoes, apples, citrus fruits, nuts (brazil nuts, almonds, walnuts), seeds (flaxseed, sunflower seeds, pine nuts, sesame seeds) **Eat less** salt, caffeine, refined carbohydrate foods (cakes, pastries), saturated fats, meat products (bacon, sausages, pâté, meat pies). Drink less alcohol

High cholesterol

Left unchecked, high blood cholesterol levels can cause arterial disease such as atherosclerosis (narrowing of the arteries), heart attacks, and strokes.
Eat more oily fish, high-fibre foods (wholegrains, oats, bran, barley, brown rice, beans, peas), olive oil, vitamin C-rich foods (kiwi fruit, citrus fruit, peppers, broccoli), vitamin E-rich foods (almonds, walnuts), seeds (sesame, pumpkin, sunflower)
Eat less saturated fats and processed foods

Insomnia

Tryptophan, a relaxing substance connected with the production of serotonin, is present in some foods and appears to encourage sleep.
Eat more tryptophan-releasing foods (chicken, turkey, pasta, rice, beans, potatoes, root vegetables, basil, lettuce, broccoli, figs, dates, bananas, hazelnuts)
Eat less high-protein foods and drink less caffeine in the evening

Irritable Bowel Syndrome (IBS)

Certain foods in certain people trigger the symptoms of IBS. Learn your triggers and avoid them. It may also help to avoid large meals.

If constipation is a symptom of your IBS:
Eat more high-fibre foods (wholegrains, oats, bran, broccoli, cabbage, beans, peas, fruit) – add these to yor diet gradually so as not to worsen wind or cramps; drink more water

If diarrhoea is a symptom of your IBS:
Eat more startchy foods (wholewheat bread and pasta, brown rice, live yoghurt

For both symptoms:
Eat less fatty and spicy foods and milk products, and drink less alcohol and caffeine

Low male fertility

Bear in mind that being overweight can also affect fertility.
Eat more vitamin C-rich foods, beta-carotene foods (orange and dark green fruit and vegetables), zinc-rich foods (such as shellfish, pumpkin seeds)
Drink less alcohol and caffeinated drinks

Menopausal problems

Eating phytoestrogen-containing foods can help correct the hormonal imbalance, though their oestrogen-like effect is weak compared to the strength of the naturally-occurring oestrogens in a woman's body.

Eat more oily fish, wholegrains, brown rice, beans, lentils, chickpeas, soya beans and soya products, alfalfa, peas, beetroot, fennel, broccoli, beetroot, celery, seeds
Eat less sugar, saturated fats; drink less coffee

Osteoarthritis

Osteo- and rheumatoid arthirtis are the two most common types of arthritis. Certain foods help halt the progression of this joint disease and deal with the pain and inflammation.
Eat more oily fish, wholegrains, beans, fresh fruit and vegetables, sweet potatoes, ginger, walnuts, chestnuts, flaxseeds
Eat less highly refined products, saturated and trans fats; drink fewer fizzy drinks

Osteoporosis

Eating bone-strengthening foods throughout your life can help prevent osteoporosis in later life or mitigate the resulting damage.
Eat more seafood, calcium- and vitamin D-rich foods (low-fat dairy products or fortified soya products), olive oil, beans, peas, green leafy vegetables, apples, flaxseed
Eat less refined sugar, salt, saturated fat. Drink less coffee, alcohol, fewer fizzy drinks

Pre-menstrual syndrome (PMS)

Cut down on refined and processed foods and eat as much freshly prepared food as possible.
Eat more oily fish, shellfish, wholegrains, oats, brown rice, soya products, beans, lentils, chickpeas, beansprouts, peas, beetroot, fennel, sweet potatoes, broccoli, brussels sprouts, rhubarb, flaxseed, sunflower seeds and pumpkin seeds
Eat less spicy foods, chocolate, cakes, biscuits, drink less coffee, alcohol

Prostate gland problems

Eating foods high in phytoestrogens may be beneficial for prostate problems.
Eat more oily fish, shellfish, eggs, soya beans and soya products, chickpeas, lentils, peas, fennel, tomatoes and tomato products, avocados, molasses, nuts, flaxseed; drink more green tea, red wine
Eat less processed foods

Rheumatoid arthritis

Improving diet may help reduce the pain and prevent some of the disability associated with this form of arthritis.
Eat more white and oily fish, eggs, olive oil, fresh fruit and vegetables, sunflower seeds
Eat less saturated fat, dairy foods, omega-6 fatty acids (polyunsaturated oils)

Stress

Diet can play a part in tackling stress (a risk factor for heart disease).
Eat more oily fish, skinless chicken, low-fat dairy products, unrefined wholefoods (wholemeal bread, pasta, rice, oats), fruit
Eat less red meat, 'junk food', sugary foods, takeaways; drink less caffeine, alcohol

the 100 foods

apples

Apples were introduced to the West by the Romans, and today there are more than 2,000 different cultivars. An apple a day really does help keep the doctor away, thanks to apples' potent **antioxidant phytochemicals**, which help protect the heart, contribute to a healthy urinary tract and healthy vision, and bolster **anti-cancer** defences.

The soluble fibre in apples, pectin, **helps lower blood cholesterol** levels, reducing the risk of heart disease. Pectin also improves the efficiency of the digestive system by removing toxic metals such as lead and mercury from the body. Apples are therefore good for a detoxification programme and especially useful if you live in traffic-heavy urban areas.

Ideal as a low-calorie snack, apples release sugar slowly into the bloodstream and are great for helping raise flagging energy levels.

✱ storing and serving Buy organic fruit whenever possible to avoid residual pesticides, and wash thoroughly. Eat unpeeled or juiced whole, including the pips, for maximum nutritional benefit. The fresher the apple the more vitamin C it contains.

baked apples with lemon

1 Core **4 large eating apples** and enlarge the holes with a small knife. Score around the middle of each apple so the skins do not burst.

2 Cut **1 lemon** lengthways into 4. Roll the lemon pieces in a mixture of **50 g (2 oz) light muscovado sugar** and **1 teaspoon ground cinnamon**. Push a coated lemon wedge into each apple cavity.

3 Bake the apples in a foil-lined dish in a preheated oven, 180°C (350°F), Gas 4, for 45 minutes. Serve with fromage frais. **serves 4**

NUTRITIONAL CONTENT PER APPLE (SMALL): energy 47 kcals | **protein** 0.4 g | **carbohydrates** 12 g | **fat** 0 g | **fibre** 2 g | **vitamin C** 6 mg | **potassium** 120 mg | **calcium** 4 mg

41

42

pears

Like apples, pears provide plenty of fibre, including the soluble fibre pectin, which helps cleanse the colon and keep it healthy, and to **lower blood cholesterol** levels, which helps protect the heart. Also, like apples, pears help rid the body of toxins, and a detoxification programme of pears alone for a day or so will deep cleanse your digestive system and benefit your skin.

Although not especially rich in nutrients, pears contain vitamins A, C, E and K and some **potassium** and copper, and their **iodine** can aid thyroid function. The protective antioxidants in pears include the flavonoid epicatechin, which helps fight the free radicals linked to the negative effects of ageing.

Canned pears are nutritionally inferior to fresh ones, containing not only between a half and two-thirds less vitamin C and fibre but also more calories.

✱ storing and serving Ripe pears do not keep well and bruise easily, so choose firm, unwrinkled fruits, preferably organic to avoid pesticide residues. Store them out of direct sunlight or in the refrigerator if they are already ripe. Eat fresh pears, with the skin, as soon as possible for maximum nutritional benefit.

pear and stilton salad

1 Core and quarter **4 pears** and slice each quarter in half. Cook the pear slices on a preheated griddle pan for 1 minute on each side. Transfer to a plate and sprinkle over **4 tablespoons lemon juice**.

2 Arrange **250 g (8 oz) baby spinach** (or mixed salad leaves) on 4 plates, arrange the griddled pears on top and sprinkle with **4 chopped walnuts, 250 g (8 oz) crumbled Stilton** and **4 tablespoons walnut oil**. Serve immediately. **serves 4**

NUTRITIONAL CONTENT PER PEAR (LARGE): energy 80 kcals | **protein** 0.3 g | **carbohydrates** 20 g | **fat** 0.2 g | **fibre** 4 g | **vitamin C** 12 mg | **potassium** 150 mg | **calcium** 22 mg

43

bananas

The high **potassium** levels in bananas means that eating them regularly can help **maintain a healthy heart**, **control blood pressure** and **promote healthy bones**. Bananas are also full of the vital antioxidants beta-carotene (the precursor to vitamin A) and vitamin C, both of which **boost the immune system** and protect against heart disease and some cancers.

The vitamin B_6 in bananas regulates the nervous system and helps promote healthy skin, while the amino acid tryptophan may help reduce symptoms of premenstrual syndrome (PMS), anxiety and insomnia.

Their high fibre content makes bananas mildly laxative, but ripe ones can help alleviate diarrhoea. A source of slow-release energy, they are great for breakfast or as a snack, and can be eaten before, during or after exercise. Dried bananas also make a good snack, with higher levels of fibre and potassium.

✱ storing and serving Choose firm yellow bananas and store them at room temperature away from other fruit because they can make them over-ripen. Although they look unappealing, browny-black bananas are ideal weaning food for babies.

banana and peanut butter smoothie

1 Peel and slice **1 ripe banana** and freeze it for at least 2 hours or overnight.

2 Put the frozen banana in a blender or food processor with **300 ml (½ pint) semi-skimmed milk** and **1 tablespoon smooth peanut butter (or 2 teaspoons tahini paste)** and process until smooth.

3 Pour into a glass and serve immediately. **serves 1**

NUTRITIONAL CONTENT PER BANANA (MEDIUM, NO SKIN): energy 95 kcals | **protein** 1.2 g | **carbohydrates** 23 g | **fat** 0.3 g | **fibre** 3 g | **vitamin C** 11 mg | **potassium** 400 mg | **calcium** 6 mg

45

NUTRITIONAL CONTENT PER 20 GRAPES: energy 60 kcals | protein 0.4 g | carbohydrates 15 g | fat 0.1 g | fibre 1 g | **vitamin C** 3 mg | potassium 210 mg | calcium 13 mg | magnesium 7 mg

grapes

Red (black) grapes and red wine have long been recognized as providing some protection against heart disease and red or purple grape juice is believed to offer the same health benefits. This is attributed to the health-boosting compounds in grapes, particularly the flavonoids quercitin and resveratrol. Resveratrol, found in red grape skins, has strong **antioxidant** and **anti-inflammatory** properties and is believed to help prevent cancer, to improve blood flow to the brain, thus reducing the risk of stroke, and to make the blood less likely to clot.

Green (white) grapes contain little or no resveratrol, but the high quantity of other antioxidants in both types of grape is believed to lower cholesterol levels, reduce the risk of cancer and boost brain power.

Raisins are grapes that have been dehydrated and are an equally rich source of antioxidants.

✱ **storing and serving** Store grapes, unwashed, in the refrigerator and keep them on their stems until required. Just before use, wash well under running water to remove pesticide residues, but don't peel or you will remove many of the important nutrients. Eat as a snack, serve with cheese or use in salads.

black grape jelly with citrus fruits

1 Gently heat **150 ml (¼ pint) red grape juice** with **2 sachets gelatine**. Allow to cool. Mix the dissolved gelatine with **450 ml (¾ pint) red grape juice**.

2 Put **175 g (6 oz) halved red and green grapes** in 4 glasses; pour over the jelly. Chill until set.

3 Segment **1 orange** and **1 pink grapefruit**, collecting the juice in a pan. Add **1 tablespoon caster sugar** and heat until dissolved. Bring to a simmer then add the segments and leave to cool.

4 To serve, spoon the citrus segments and a little juice on the jelly. **serves 4**

grapefruit

Grapefruit help promote a healthy heart, being a rich source of vitamin C and bioflavonoids, which protect the arteries and improve blood circulation. **Folic acid** and **potassium** further help protect the heart.

Grapefruit also have **anti-cancer** properties. Pink and red types have a significant quantity of **lycopene**, believed to reduce the risk of prostate cancer. They also contain a number of other cancer-inhibiting compounds, including **limonene**, found in all citrus oils, that may help reduce tumour growth.

The bitter-tasting flavonoid compound **naringin**, thought to inhibit the uptake of fatty acids into cells thus preventing the body from using carbohydrates effectively, makes grapefruit good for weight loss.

Grapefruit pectin, the soluble fibre found in the white pith between segments, is good for **lowering blood cholesterol levels** and detoxifying.

✱ storing and serving Grapefruit can be left in the fruit bowl for a week or in the refrigerator for several weeks. Bring to room temperature before use because the fruit is at its juiciest when slightly warm.

pink grapefruit and pine nut salad

1 Peel and segment **2 pink grapefruit**, working over a dish to collect the juice.

2 Halve, stone and peel **2 avocados**. Slice the flesh and mix with the reserved citrus juice.

3 Lightly toast **75 g (3 oz) pine nuts** under a grill or dry-fry them in a frying pan. Sprinkle the nuts over the avocado and grapefruit and offer grated **Parmesan** separately. **serves 4**

NUTRITIONAL CONTENT PER GRAPEFRUIT (MEDIUM): energy 105 kcals **| protein** 4 g **| carbohydrates** 25 g **| fat** 0 g **| fibre** 10 g **| vitamin C** 126 mg **| potassium** 700 mg **| calcium** 8 mg

49

lemons and limes

The health-boosting powers of lemons and limes have long been known. In the 18th century British sailors were given a ration of lime juice every day to prevent scurvy (a deficiency disease caused by lack of vitamin C); this earned them their nickname 'limeys'.

Like all citrus fruit, lemons and limes contain loads of **vitamin C**, which helps white blood cells fight infection, boosts immunity in general and helps maintain mental alertness and a retentive memory. It is also needed for healing wounds and may help reduce some of the symptoms of arthritis.

Other antioxidants in citrus fruit, bioflavonoids, work with vitamin C to strengthen blood vessel walls, reducing the risk of stroke and heart disease. Studies suggest that the citrus oil **limonene** can reduce the growth of cancerous tumours and possibly **lower blood cholesterol**.

✻ **storing and serving** Lemons will keep for a week or two at room temperature and for longer if refrigerated. Limes are best kept in the refrigerator. You will get the most juice from the fruit if you bring it to room temperature and roll it on a flat surface before squeezing.

lemon and basil penne

1 Cook **175 g (6 oz) dried penne** in boiling water according to the instructions on the packet.

2 Meanwhile, blend together **2 garlic cloves**, a large **handful of basil leaves, 4 tablespoons olive oil** and the grated rind and juice of **2 lemons**. Add **50 g (2 oz) grated Parmesan** and season with **pepper** to taste.

3 Drain the pasta, stir through the pesto and serve immediately. **serves 4**

oranges

Oranges are known for their high vitamin C content, which is important for a **healthy immune system** and helps the body disarm the cell-damaging free radicals that accelerate ageing and cause diseases such as cancer, heart disease and strokes.

Oranges are packed with plenty of other health-boosters, including fibre, which helps **keep cholesterol levels down** and the digestive system operating efficiently, and powerful **flavonoids**, like herperidin, which is even more effective than vitamin C in fighting high cholesterol levels, high blood pressure and other factors implicated in diseases.

Research has linked a citrus-rich diet with a reduced risk of certain cancers. This is due to a compound found citrus oils called **limonene**, which is believed to reduce the growth of tumours.

✱ storing and serving Oranges can be stored at room temperature or in the refrigerator. Most of the potent phytonutrients are found in the peel (and the oil it contains), so use the rind whenever possible in baking and desserts. However, avoid using fruit that has been waxed to improve its appearance.

carrot soup with orange and ginger

1 Peel and roughly chop **750 g (1½ lb) carrots** and finely chop a **5 cm (2 inch) piece of fresh root ginger**. Add to a saucepan containing **900 ml (1½ pints) vegetable stock (or water)**. Bring to the boil, then simmer for 12–15 minutes or until cooked through.

2 Stir **2 tablespoons chopped parsley** into the soup and process in batches with **150 ml (¼ pint) orange juice**. Season to taste with **salt and pepper**.

3 Return to the pan, simmer gently to reheat and serve with a little **buttermilk (or natural yogurt)** swirled on top. **serves 6**

NUTRITIONAL CONTENT PER 100G ORANGE (PEELED): energy 34 kcals | **protein** 1.1 g | **carbohydrates** 9 g | **fat** 0.1 g | **fibre** 2 g | **vitamin C** 54 mg | **potassium** 150 mg | **calcium** 47 mg

53

NUTRITIONAL CONTENT PER 100 G: energy 36 kcals | protein 0.5 g | **carbohydrates** 9 g | **fat** 0 g | **fibre** 2 g | **vitamin C** 60 mg | **potassium** 200 mg | **calcium** 23 mg | **magnesium** 11 mg | **iron** 0.5 mg

papayas

Containing more vitamin C and **potassium** than oranges, papayas are **nutritional superfoods**. They are packed with cholesterol-lowering fibre and with antioxidants, including the eye-saving carotenoids lutein and zeaxanthin; lycopene, which is linked with prostate health; and the phytochemicals carpaine and cryptoxanthin, which are believed to help protect from cancer.

The high levels of beta-carotene (which the body converts to vitamin A) and vitamin C work together, making this tropical fruit great for the **immune system**. They also help maintain healthy skin by encouraging elasticity, hindering the formation of wrinkles and keeping skin cells plump.

Papayas are great for detoxifying the body. They contain papain, a digestive enzyme that helps break down protein and cleanse the digestive tract, which can, in turn, help with weight loss.

✱ **storing and serving** Papayas are best when ripe. They should have a strong fragrance, and the skin should be firm but yield to pressure. Leave them in the fruit bowl to ripen then store in the refrigerator and eat within a day or two. Halve lengthways, scoop out the seeds and eat the flesh with a spoon.

grilled fruit

1 Halve **1 large papaya**, remove the seeds then peel and slice the flesh. Peel and slice the flesh from **1 large mango**. Peel and cut **2 bananas** in half and slice the pieces in half lengthways. Peel and thinly slice **2 oranges**.

2 Arrange the fruit in a foil-lined grill pan and dot with **25 g (1 oz) unsalted butter**. Sprinkle with **40 g (1½ oz) brown sugar** and cook under a hot grill for 10–15 minutes, turning occasionally and basting with the melted sugar, butter and fruit juices. Serve with **natural yogurt. serves 4**

figs

Figs are good for the digestive system. They are packed with fibre and also contain ficin, an enzyme that helps soothe the gut. They are mildly laxative.

Figs contain compounds that help shrink tumours and are, therefore, believed to help prevent cancer. They are also one of the highest plant sources of **calcium**, which is required for good bone health, blood clotting and healthy nerve function.

The other nutrients in figs, including **iron** and **potassium**, are particularly concentrated in dried figs, which provide instant energy and help prevent cramps, so making them ideal for athletes. The amino acid tryptophan makes figs a natural sedative.

Figs appear to trigger headaches in some people. The oxalates in them make them unsuitable for people suffering from kidney or gallbladder problems.

✱ storing and serving Keep under-ripe figs at room temperature out of direct sunlight. Store ripe figs in the refrigerator but bring to room temperature to serve. Use fresh figs raw as a snack, serve them in salads or with cheese or poach them for desserts. Use dried figs in breakfast cereals and baking.

fig, mozzarella and prosciutto salad

1 Cut **8 ripe black figs** into quarters and tear **250 g (8 oz) mozzarella** and **8 slices prosciutto** into bite-size pieces. Arrange them all on a large platter with a few **basil leaves**.

2 Whisk together **3 tablespoons olive oil, 1 tablespoon white wine vinegar** and a **pinch of sugar**.

3 Season the dressing with **salt and pepper** and drizzle over the salad. **serves 4**

NUTRITIONAL CONTENT PER 100 G FRESH (DRIED): energy 43 (227) kcals I **protein** 1.3 (3.6) g I **carbohydrates** 10 (53) g I **fat** 0.3 (1.6) g I **fibre** 2 (12) g I **vitamin C** 2 (1) mg I **potassium** 200 (970) mg

57

mangoes

Another orange-coloured fruit with plenty of beta-carotene (the precursor to vitamin A in the body), the mango is similar to the papaya with its package of antioxidant and detoxifying phytonutrients.

Mangoes have powerful **immunity-boosting properties** thanks to the antioxidant vitamins A, C and E they contain. These roam the body, neutralizing the cell-damaging free radicals responsible for premature ageing and degenerative diseases such as clogged arteries, strokes, heart disease and cancer.

Packed with soluble fibre, which has cholesterol-removing properties, and insoluble fibre, which helps maintain bowel health, mangoes are also good for the digestive system and useful for soothing indigestion.

The detoxifying properties of mangoes mean they are good for cleansing the kidneys and blood and can help improve skin texture.

✱ storing and serving A ripe mango is firm to the touch but with a little 'give'. Leave under-ripe fruit in the fruit bowl to ripen, then refrigerate. Add mangoes to smoothies for the flavour, although the thick juice is best thinned with apple or pear juice.

mango, avocado and chicken

1 Halve, stone and peel **2 ripe avocados**. Dice the flesh and transfer to a shallow bowl with **2 tablespoons lemon juice**.

2 Peel, stone and dice the flesh of **1 small mango**.

3 Mix **3 tablespoons olive oil, 1 teaspoon wholegrain mustard, 1 teaspoon clear honey, 2 teaspoons cider vinegar** and **salt and pepper**. Add the lemon juice from the avocado.

4 Arrange **50 g (2 oz) sliced cooked beetroot** and a handful of **watercress** in a bowl and add the avocado and mango. Add the dressing and **175 g (6 oz) thinly sliced smoked chicken. serves 4**

NUTRITIONAL CONTENT PER 100 G: energy 57 kcals | **protein** 0.7 g | **carbohydrates** 14 g | **fat** 0.2 g | **fibre** 3 g | **vitamin C** 37 mg | **carotene** 1800 mcg | **potassium** 180 mg | **calcium** 12 mg

59

apricots

Apricots are rich in beta-carotene, which offers some protection against cancer and eye problems, such as cataracts, by neutralizing the free radicals that damage body cells and tissues. Beta-carotene and lycopene, another antioxidant present, also help prevent the formation of plaque in arteries, which can result in high blood pressure and heart disease.

Fresh apricots are rich in vitamin C, and they help regulate the digestive system, being especially helpful in relieving constipation. The soluble fibre pectin also helps to **lower blood cholesterol**.

Dried apricots have an increased concentration of beta-carotene, **iron**, **potassium**, **calcium** and magnesium. Iron is needed to form haemoglobin in blood cells, potassium benefits blood pressure, and calcium and magnesium are needed for strong healthy bones and to help prevent osteoporosis.

✷ **choosing dried apricots** Avoid dried apricots preserved with sulphur dioxide as this can trigger asthma attacks. Any pesticide residues are more concentrated in the dried fruit, so choose organic brands, especially for children.

poached apricots with oatmeal cream

1 Heat **2 tablespoons light muscovado sugar**, ½ **teaspoon ground ginger** and **5 tablespoons water** until the sugar has dissolved.

2 Quarter and pit **500 g (1 lb) fresh apricots**, add to the pan, cover and simmer gently for about 10 minutes. Cool slightly.

3 Meanwhile, dry-fry **40 g (1½ oz) oatmeal** for about 30 seconds. Cool slightly, then stir into **200 g (7 oz) Greek yogurt** and **2 tablespoons double cream** and **2 tablespoons honey**. Spoon over the apricots and serve. **serves 4**

NUTRITIONAL CONTENT PER 100 G FRESH (DRIED): **energy** 29 (158) kcals I **protein** 1 (4) g I **carbohydrates** 7 (37) g I **fat** 0 (1) g I **fibre** 2 (18) g I **vitamin** 5 (1) mg I **potassium** 250 (1380) mg

61

NUTRITIONAL CONTENT PER 100 G: energy 40 kcals | protein 1.1 g | carbohydrates 11 g |
fat 0.5 g | fibre 2 g | vitamin C 59 mg | potassium 290 mg | calcium 25 mg | magnesium 15 mg

kiwi fruit

Kiwi fruit, once known as Chinese gooseberries, are packed with antioxidants including high levels of vitamins C and E; kiwi fruit actually contain more vitamin C than oranges – so eating kiwi fruit can help boost immunity and ward off cancer, heart disease and other degenerative diseases and conditions. They can also help the body deal with stress. Another antioxidant, lutein, helps maintain healthy vision. Kiwi fruit also contain **potassium**, needed for healthy blood pressure, and **folic acid**, important before and during pregnancy to protect against birth defects.

Current research shows that kiwi fruit can help with respiratory-related disorders and may provide an alternative to aspirin for thinning the blood to reduce the risk of clots and protect cardiovascular health.

Kiwi fruit are also a good source of digestive enzymes, including atinidin, which aid digestion.

✱ **storing and serving** Ripe kiwi fruit will keep in the refrigerator for one to two weeks. Store them away from other fruit that emit ethylene gas, which will over-ripen the kiwi fruit. To serve, cut the peeled fruit into slices or wedges, or cut the top off the unpeeled fruit like a boiled egg and eat with a spoon.

kiwi fruit, melon and grape salad

1 Cut a thin slice from the base of **1 large Galia melon**, slice off the top and discard the seeds. Scoop the flesh into small balls. Reserve the shell.

2 Skin **125 (4 oz) seedless green grapes**, thinly slice **3 kiwi fruit** and peel, core and thinly slice **2 apples**. Put the fruit in a bowl with the melon balls and a drained **325 g (11 oz) can lychees**. Sprinkle with **3 tablespoons kirsch**, cover and chill until ready to serve.

3 Put the melon shell on a serving plate, pile the fruit into the shell and decorate with **mint sprigs**. **serves 4–6**

63

guavas

Guavas are tropical fruit with edible skin and seeds and a pungent fragrance. They are a **top antioxidant fruit**, containing more vitamin C and more lycopene than probably any other known fruit or vegetable, and the red- or pink-fleshed guavas are especially high in lycopene. Guavas are also rich in beta-carotene (the precursor to vitamin A in the body) and soluble fibre. These four nutrients, plus others including **potassium** help maintain healthy **blood cholesterol levels** and blood pressure levels and account for guavas' outstanding contribution to heart health.

As well as boosting heart health, lycopene (the same antioxidant carotenoid that gives the red colour to tomatoes and watermelon) is also believed to help prevent cancer, particularly prostate cancer.

In addition, guavas are thought to have **anti-microbial** properties and are used in the tropics to treat diarrhoea.

✳ storing and serving Because vitamin C reduces with each day of storage, look for unblemished fruit when buying and eat as soon as possible after purchase. Eat guavas fresh as long as they are very ripe or use them in jams, fruit salad and desserts, such as custards and ice cream.

guava, apple and banana smoothie

1 Peel, halve and deseed **2 ripe guavas** and roughly chop the flesh. Peel, core and roughly chop **1 apple** and thickly slice **2 bananas**. Process the fruit together until smooth.

2 Add **125 g (4 oz) raspberries (or strawberries)** together with **200 ml (7 fl oz) natural yogurt** and **150 ml (¼ pint) cold water**. Process again until smooth. Pour over ice cubes and drink immediately. **serves 4**

NUTRITIONAL CONTENT PER 100 G FLESH: energy 41 kcals | protein 0.4 g | carbohydrates 10 g | fat 0.2 g | fibre 1 g | vitamin C 12 mg | potassium 160 mg | calcium 18 mg | magnesium 16 mg

pineapples

Eating pineapple can aid digestion and help reduce inflammation due to the high levels of the enzyme bromelain. This acts by digesting protein, making it helpful for **clearing a sluggish digestive system**, and by breaking down areas of inflamed body tissue, thus making pineapple useful for sufferers of osteoarthritis, gout, hay fever and asthma. Eating pineapple on its own between meals maximizes bromelain's **anti-inflammatory** effect. Bromelain also helps prevent blood clots and promotes the healing of minor injuries, and has **anti-cancer** properties.

Pineapples are rich in beta-carotene and vitamin C, two of the many antioxidants that protect the body from free radicals that cause degenerative diseases.

The vitamin B1 in pineapple helps energy production, the **potassium** helps regulate blood pressure, while the high manganese content helps protect against hardening of the arteries and is vital for forming bones and cartilage and for maintaining a good **immune system**.

✱ **storing and serving** A pineapple will not ripen once picked, so check your pineapple is ripe – there should be a sweet smell at the stem end. Add fresh pineapple to salads and salsa or griddle for dessert.

baked pineapple rings with cinnamon

1 Peel and core **1 small pineapple** and cut it into 1 cm (½ inch) rings. Pat them dry on kitchen paper.

2 Combine **50 g (2 oz) dark muscovado sugar, 1 teaspoon ground cinnamon** and a **pinch of mild chilli powder** in a plastic bag. Add the pineapple rings and toss well to coat.

3 Arrange the pineapple on a foil-lined baking sheet, dust with **caster sugar** and bake in a preheated oven, 200°C (400°F), Gas 6, for 20 minutes. Serve with **fromage frais**. **serves 4**

pomegranates

Recent studies of the health-boosting properties of the **antioxidant-rich** pomegranate suggest that the antioxidant action of its juice is three times more potent than a similar quantity of red wine or green tea, so a daily glass may reduce the risk of heart disease thanks to its tannins, polyphenols, and anthocyanidins, which work by improving the function of blood vessels and reducing hardening of the arteries, as well as **reducing blood cholesterol levels** and high blood pressure. Research suggests that a daily glass is also great for prostate health and may slow the growth of prostate and other tumours, thanks to the high levels of **flavonoids** (antioxidants that are effective at disarming free radicals).

The phyto-oestrogens (natural oestrogen) in pomegranates mean they may also be useful for treating some symptoms of the menopause.

✱ storing and serving Keep pomegranates in the refrigerator for up to three months; at room temperature they will last only two to three days. Use the pulp and seeds in salads and relishes; use the fruit in drinks and sauces.

pomegranate and mixed-leaf salad

1 Put **3 tablespoons raspberry vinegar** and **2 tablespoons olive oil** in a salad bowl, season with **salt and pepper** and mix lightly.

2 Cut **1 pomegranate** in half, break or cut it into large pieces and flex the skin so that the seeds fall out. Pick out and discard any stubborn seeds. Add the remainder to the salad bowl, discarding the skin and pith.

3 Toss **125 g (4 oz) mixed salad leaves** (including baby spinach leaves, red mustard and mizuna) in the dressing, tearing large leaves into bite-sized pieces. Serve sprinkled with **fresh raspberries**, if liked. **serves 6**

NUTRITIONAL CONTENT PER 100 G FLESH: energy 72 kcals | **protein** 1 g | **carbohydrates** 17 g | **fat** 1 g | **fibre** 1 g | **vitamin C** 7 mg | **potassium** 379 mg | **calcium** 13 mg | **magnesium** 12 mg

69

blueberries

Try to eat a handful a day of these antioxidant foods. Blueberries are **packed with anthocyanidins**, which help fight infection and inflammation. They neutralize harmful free radicals and help maintain a healthy vascular system, protecting against varicose veins, heart disease, haemorrhoids and hardening of the arteries.

Anthocyanidins in blueberries may slow and even **reverse age-related mental decline**, and lessen brain damage inflicted by strokes.

Blueberries also contain pterostilbene, which fights cancer, and the soluble fibre pectin, which is thought to help prevent cancer; both compounds help **reduce blood cholesterol** levels. Blueberries also benefit night vision and can help treat diarrhoea and constipation.

Unrelated to blueberries but similar in appearance, **açaí berries** are thought to be even higher in antioxidants than blueberries and are one of the most nutritious and powerful foods in the world. They are currently the subject of much research.

✳ storing and serving Blueberries should be eaten fresh or frozen on the day of purchase.

blueberry and raspberry brûlée

1 Arrange a mixture of **250 g (8 oz) blueberries** and **250 g (8 oz) raspberries** in 4 heatproof dishes.

2 Spoon **350 g (12 oz) fromage frais** over the fruit and smooth the surface.

3 Sprinkle **4–6 tablespoons soft dark brown sugar** evenly over the top and cook under a preheated hot grill, close to the heat, for 1–2 minutes or until the sugar has melted and is bubbling. **serves 4**

NUTRITIONAL CONTENT PER 100 G: energy 57 kcals I **protein** 1 g I **carbohydrates** 15 g I **fat** 0.3 g I **fibre** 2 g I **vitamin C** 10 mg I **potassium** 77 mg I **calcium** 6 mg I **magnesium** 6 mg

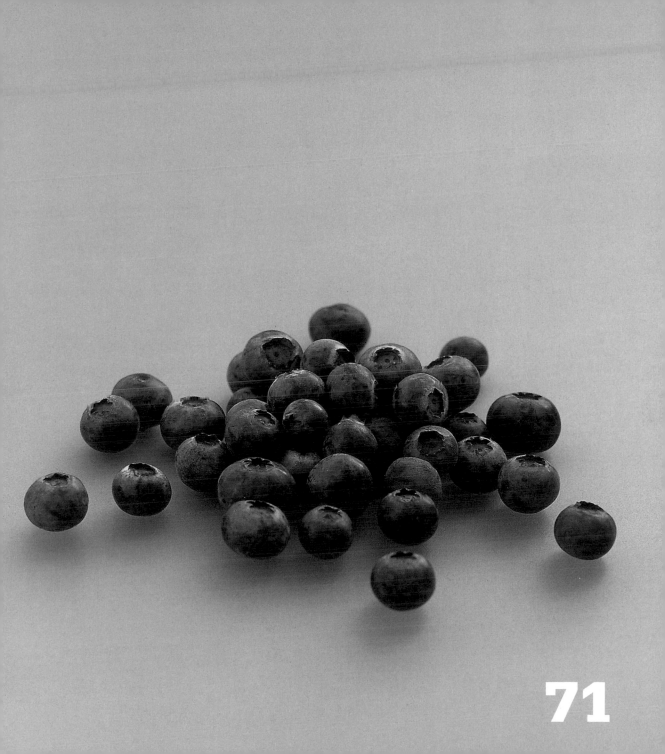

raspberries

All berries are brimming with the vitamins and antioxidants that help protect against premature ageing and diseases such as cancer. In raspberries the health-boosting antioxidant phytonutrients include **ellagic acid**, which may help prevent the growth of cancerous cells, and a group of flavonoids called anthocyanidins, which have **antimicrobial** properties and can prevent the overgrowth of certain fungi and bacteria in the body, like the yeast *Candida albicans*, which causes thrush.

Raspberries also help reduce the risk of coronary heart disease. Their fibre content helps lower the levels of 'bad' cholesterol in the body, while their antioxidants help decrease the build-up of 'bad' cholesterol on artery walls.

Mildy laxative, raspberries are good for indigestion and can help alleviate diarrhoea. They are also effective for menstrual and menopausal problems.

✱ storing and serving Raspberries are highly perishable, so store in the refrigerator and use within a day or two. They freeze well – use frozen berries within a year.

raspberry and passionfruit fool

1 Whip together **200 ml (7 fl oz) evaporated milk** and **1 tablespoon caster sugar** until the mixture is thick and fluffy.

2 Process **225 g (7½ oz) raspberries** until smooth, then stir into the whipped evaporated milk with **225 g (7½ oz) whole raspberries** and the flesh of **2 passionfruits**. Spoon into serving dishes and serve. **serves 4**

NUTRITIONAL CONTENT PER 100 G: **energy** 25 kcals | **protein** 1 g |**carbohydrates** 5 g | **fat** 0 g | **fibre** 7 g | **vitamin C** 32 mg | **potassium** 170 mg | **calcium** 25 mg | **magnesium** 19 mg

blackberries

Like raspberries, blackberries contain anthocyanidins, which have strong antioxidant and **anti-inflammatory** properties. Their high tannin content gives them an astringent action so they can neutralize excessive acid in the body, helping to relieve joint pains. They help sore throats and chesty coughs and help clear diarrhoea and urinary tract infections.

Rich in **vitamin E**, blackberries promote a healthy heart and good circulation. They also boost the blood, and help prevent anaemia. Pectin, the soluble fibre in blackberries, helps **reduce blood cholesterol** levels, thereby reducing the risk of heart disease and stroke.

The aspirin-like compounds in blackberries, salicylates, are thought to lower the risk of heart problems, but if you are intolerant of aspirin you may have an allergic reaction to blackberries.

✱ storing and serving Choose shiny berries with a rich aroma and use them as soon as possible, washing them just before use. Blackberries freeze well; open-freeze on trays then bag and seal – keep for up to six months.

blackberry and oat layer

1 Spread **25 g (1 oz) oats** with **2 tablespoons clear honey** on a baking sheet. Cook in a preheated oven, 180°C (350°F), Gas Mark 4, for 10–15 minutes, stirring twice.

2 Remove from the oven, add **15 g (½ oz) chopped stem ginger** and leave to cool. Stir the oats to break up any large lumps.

3 Roughly crush **175 g (6 oz) blackberries**. Mix **150 ml (¼ pint) natural yogurt** and **150 ml (¼ pint) crème fraîche** and the **grated rind of ½ lemon**. Stir in **1 tablespoon clear honey**.

4 Layer the blackberries and oats with the yogurt mixture in 4 glasses. Chill for 1–2 hours. **serves 4**

NUTRITIONAL CONTENT PER 100 G: energy 25 kcals | **protein** 0.9 g | **carbohydrates** 5 g | **fat** 0.2 g | **fibre** 7 g | **vitamin C** 15 mg | **vitamin E** 2.37 mg | **potassium** 160 mg | **calcium** 41 mg

strawberries

A daily portion of strawberries can help ward off infections and keep your heart healthy by raising blood folate levels, which helps to reduce the build-up of the harmful amino acid homocysteine in the blood, and by reducing systolic blood pressure. Strawberries may also be anti-ageing.

The fruits have some of the same disease-fighting antioxidants as raspberries, including ellagic acid, which combats carcinogens, and anthocyanidins, which have **anti-cancer**, **anti-microbial** and **anti-inflammatory** properties. Their antioxidant phenols may help ease arthritis and asthma, while the proanthocyanidins are thought to help keep the urinary tract and the heart healthy.

High levels of dietary fibre mean that strawberries are good for cleansing the digestive system and can reduce the risk of intestinal disorders as well as high blood pressure, diabetes and heart disease.

✱ **storing and serving** For the best flavour buy strawberries in season rather than those imported from abroad and use them as soon as possible. Wash before hulling to prevent saturating their insides.

strawberry and cucumber salad

1 Halve **1 cucumber** lengthways, remove the seeds and slice thinly. Place in a bowl with **250 g (8 oz) strawberries**, hulled and halved or quartered if large.

2 Mix together **1 tablespoon balsamic vinegar**, **1 teaspoon coarse-grain mustard**, **1 teaspoon clear honey** and **3 tablespoons olive oil**. Season with **pepper**. Pour over the cucumber and strawberries.

3 Toss lightly to coat with the dressing and chill for 5–10 minutes before serving.
serves 4–6

NUTRITIONAL CONTENT PER 100 G: **energy** 27 kcals | **protein** 1 g | **carbohydrates** 6 g | **fat** 0 g | **fibre** 2 g | **vitamin C** 77 mg | **potassium** 160 mg | **calcium** 16 mg | **magnesium** 10 mg | **iron** 0.4 mg

NUTRITIONAL CONTENT PER 100 G: energy 28 kcals | protein 1 g | carbohydrates 7 g | fat 0 g | fibre 8 g | vitamin C 200 mg | potassium 370 mg | calcium 60 mg | magnesium 17 mg | iron 1.3 mg

blackcurrants

Blackcurrants are one of the **richest sources of vitamin C** and canned blackcurrants contain nearly as much vitamin C as fresh ones.

A general immunity-boosting nutrient, vitamin C also helps protect against strokes, heart disease and cancer. The bioflavonoids in the fruit support the production of vitamin C, and these compounds work together to improve poor circulation and protect arterial health, thus helping maintain a healthy heart.

Blackcurrants are powerful antioxidants and have **anti-inflammatory** and **anti-microbial** qualities, so can help protect heart health, soothe kidney and bladder infections, and ward off cold sores and flu. They also have anti-laxative properties. Research suggests that the anthocyanidins and polyphenols may also help protect against Alzheimer's disease.

Closely related to blackcurrants, **redcurrants** contain a good amount of the antioxidant anthocyanidins but much less vitamin C. Redcurrants are believed to help with arthritis, cystitis and constipation and are great for cleansing the blood.

✱ **storing and serving** Add fresh currants to fruit salads or use them in jellies, jams and preserves. They freeze well and can be used in juices.

blackcurrant water ice

1 Put **500 g (1 lb) blackcurrants** in a pan with **2 tablespoons water**. Simmer until tender. Sieve to make 300 ml (½ pint) purée.

2 Gently heat **125 g (4 oz) caster sugar** in **150 ml (¼ pint) water**, stirring until dissolved. Bring to the boil and simmer for 5 minutes. Allow to cool. Add the syrup to the purée with **2 tablespoons lemon juice**. Tip into a freezerproof container, cover, seal and freeze.

3 When half-frozen, fold in **1 lightly whisked egg white**. Freeze until firm. Transfer to the refrigerator 15 minutes before serving to soften. **serves 4**

cranberries

Cranberries are **antioxidant powerhouses**; their phytonutrients help promote good heart health, inhibit cancerous cell growth and counter premature ageing.

A number of compounds peculiar to cranberries, including some of their proanthocyanidins, are responsible for the unique role of this fruit in **keeping the urinary system healthy**. They combat bacteria and viruses in the kidneys, bladder and urinary tract by preventing bacteria such as *E. coli* from adhering to the walls of the urinary tract, so they are ideal for people with urinary problems such as cystitis.

Similar anti-adhesion activity elsewhere in the body accounts for the effectiveness of cranberries in preventing listeria and *Helicobacter pylori* from causing gastrointestinal problems and oral bacteria from causing tooth decay. Cranberries can also help chesty coughs and sore throats.

✱ storing and serving Fresh cranberries will last for about two weeks in the refrigerator. Frozen fruit will keep for a year. Too sharp to eat raw, cranberries are ideal combined with naturally sweeter fruits, such as apples, and cooked to make jams and sauces.

cranberry muffins

1 Beat together **1 egg**, **100 ml (3½ fl oz) milk** and **75 g (3 oz) softened unsalted butter**.

2 Sift together **150 g (5 oz) plain flour** and **3 teaspoons baking powder** and stir into the mixture with **100 g (3½ oz) caster sugar**. Partially thaw **75 g (3 oz) frozen cranberries** and stir in.

3 Spoon into a greased and lined 15-section muffin tin. Sprinkle **2 tablespoons caster sugar** and **1 teaspoon ground cinnamon** over the muffins. Bake in a preheated oven, 180°C (350°F), Gas Mark 4, for 20 minutes. Leave to cool in the tin for 2–3 minutes, then serve at once. **makes 15**

NUTRITIONAL CONTENT PER 100 G: energy 15 kcals I **protein** 0.4 g I **carbohydrates** 3 g I **fat** 0 g I **fibre** 4 g I **vitamin C** 13 mg I **potassium** 95 mg I **calcium** 12 mg I **magnesium** 7 mg I **iron** 0.7 mg

82

cherries

Like all berries, cherries are a good source of antioxidants, particularly the anthocyanidins.

As well as helping **prevent or repair the damage done by free radicals**, the flavonoids in cherries help joint health. Research shows that these antioxidants inhibit inflammation-causing enzymes and reduce the levels of uric acid in painful joints. Eating cherries daily can help alleviate inflammatory disorders such as gout and rheumatoid arthritis as well as relieving headaches and migraine. Cherries contain several **anti-cancer** compounds, including ellagic acid.

Melatonin, a hormone produced in the brain's pineal gland and also found in significant quantities in cherries, may prevent or reduce age-related brain deterioration. Melatonin also aids the body's natural sleep patterns and may help deal with insomnia.

Cherries have a very low glycaemic index, so a handful of cherries is an ideal snack, stabilizing blood sugar levels and keeping hunger at bay.

✱ storing and serving Choose fruit on the stem to discourage decay and refrigerate for up to a week. Canned and bottled cherries retain many nutrients.

cherry clafoutis

1 Make a batter by mixing together **75 g (3 oz) plain flour, 25 g (1 oz) caster sugar, 3 eggs, 225 ml (7½ fl oz) milk** and a **few drops of vanilla extract**.

2 Grease a 1.5–1.8 litre (2½–3 pint) soufflé dish with **15 g (½ oz) butter**, heat for a few minutes, then add **500 g (1 lb) pitted black cherries** together with any juice. Cover with the batter.

3 Bake the clafoutis in a preheated oven, 200°C (400°F), Gas Mark 6, for 30 minutes or until well risen. Dust with **icing sugar** and serve at once. **serves 4**

NUTRITIONAL CONTENT PER 100 G WITH STONES: energy 39 kcals | **protein** 1 g | **carbohydrates** 10 g | **fat** 0 g | **fibre** 1 g | **vtamin C** 9 mg| **potassium** 170 mg | **calcium** 11 mg

plums and prunes

Fresh and dried plums (prunes), contain many of the disease-protective phytonutrients that help neutralize the damaging free radicals related to accelerated ageing and DNA degradation. They are also rich in **potassium**, essential for maintaining normal blood pressure and heart function and the growth and repair of lean body tissue.

Converting plums into prunes concentrates the nutrients in the dried fruit; prunes are thought to have **more than twice the antioxidant power** of the 'superfood' blueberries. The high fibre content of prunes and a bowel-stimulating chemical called hydroxyphenylisatin account for their laxative qualities and their role in reducing the risk of cancers, particularly of the bowel. The fibre in prunes is good for cholesterol levels, which maintains heart health.

Like all dried fruit, prunes boost energy. They also contain boron, which benefits menopausal women.

✽ **storing and serving** Don't avoid fresh plums with a slight whitish bloom – this is a good indicator that the fruit has not been overhandled. Let plums ripen in the fruit bowl, then refrigerate.

hot fruit salad

1 Leave **150 g (5 oz) prunes**, **150 g (5 oz) dried figs** and **175 g (6 oz) dried apricots** to soak in **600 ml (1 pint) apple juice** overnight.

2 Transfer to a saucepan and simmer for 10–15 minutes.

3 Turn into a bowl and pour over **2 tablespoons Calvados** (or brandy), if liked. Sprinkle with **25 g (1 oz) coarsely chopped walnuts** and serve with **natural yogurt**, if liked. **serves 6**

NUTRITIONAL CONTENT PER 100 G PLUMS WITH STONES (PRUNES NO STONES):
energy 34 (140) kcals | **protein** 1 (3) g | **carbohydrates** 8 (34) g | **fat** 0 (0) g | **fibre** 2 (13) g | **iron** 0.4 (2.6) mg

85

dates

Dates, especially dried ones, are a particularly sweet and satisfying food thanks to their natural sugar and fibre content. The fibre moderates the speed at which energy from the sugars is released, so that dates make a **good energizing food** for snacks and for eating both before and after exercise. The fibre content also gives dates laxative properties, while the natural sugars have a soothing influence by helping to raise levels of the calming serotonin in the brain.

Dates contain beta-carotene, vitamins B_6 and B_3 (**niacin**), which help maintain healthy skin and the nervous and digestive systems. The niacin makes dates good for those suffering from depression.

The **iron** in dates means they are useful for anyone suffering fatigue or anaemia. Dates also contain some **potassium**, which helps regulate blood pressure, and magnesium, vital for bones, muscles and the heart.

✱ storing and serving Dates are available both fresh and dried, with or without stones. Keep them in sealed plastic bags or airtight containers in the refrigerator. Some fresh dates will keep for several months, and dried dates can be kept for up to a year.

date and orange fool

1 Squeeze the juice from **2 large oranges** and make up the quantity to 275 ml (9 fl oz) with water. Place in a pan with **125 g (4 oz) stoned dates**. Bring to the boil, cover and simmer for 10 minutes or until soft.

2 Cool slightly then process in a blender until smooth. Set aside until cold.

3 Put alternate spoonfuls of date purée and **300 ml (½ pint) natural yogurt** in 4 small dishes. Swirl together attractively with a small knife.

4 Chill until required, then serve topped with **sliced banana**. **serves 4**

NUTRITIONAL CONTENT PER 100 G DRIED DATES WITH STONES: energy 227 kcals | protein 3 g | carbohydrates 57 g | fat 0 g | fibre 7 g | potassium 590 mg | calcium 38 mg

87

watermelons

The red flesh is a clue that watermelon is a rich source of lycopene, the antioxidant carotenoid that is found in tomatoes and is believed to reduce the risk of several cancers, particularly prostate cancer.

Like cantaloupe melons, watermelons are **high in vitamin C and beta-carotene** (vitamin A). The action of these antioxidants in disarming the dangerous free radicals that roam the body causing damage and premature ageing helps protect against stroke, certain cancers and heart disease. They also help maintain youthful-looking skin and encourage a **healthy immune system** and good vision; they have **anti-inflammatory** properties and may help alleviate some symptoms of asthma and rheumatoid arthritis.

The **potassium** in watermelons helps regulate blood pressure, and to maintain the body's fluid balance. Like all melons, watermelons are natural diuretics and a good choice for anyone suffering water retention.

✱ storing and serving A whole watermelon can be stored at room temperature if it's not too warm, but it is best refrigerated. Once cut open, refrigerate watermelon wrapped tightly in plastic.

watermelon and feta salad

1 Dry-fry **1 tablespoon black sesame seeds** for a few minutes until aromatic.

2 Arrange **500 g (1 lb) peeled and diced watermelon** and **175 g (6 oz) diced feta cheese** on a plate with **50 g (2 oz) rocket leaves** and a few **herb sprigs**.

3 Whisk **6 tablespoons olive oil**, **1 tablespoon pomegranate syrup, 1 tablespoon orange flower juice, 1½ tablespoons lemon juice** and **½ teaspoon sugar**. Season with **salt and pepper** and drizzle over the salad. Scatter over the sesame seeds and serve with toasted **pitta bread**. **serves 4 as a starter**

NUTRITIONAL CONTENT PER 100 G FLESH: energy 31 kcals | protein 1 g | carbohydrates 7 g | fat 0 g | fibre 0 g | vitamin C 8 mg | potassium 100 mg | magnesium 8 mg

89

cantaloupe melons

These orange-fleshed melons, also known as musk melons, are excellent sources of beta-carotene and vitamin C. These nutrients are **powerful antioxidants**, which neutralize the free radicals that cause heart disease, cancer and premature ageing. In addition, they help maintain healthy, youthful skin by encouraging skin cell turnover and maintaining the elasticity and plumpness of the skin. Beta-carotene may also provide protection from within against damage to the skin from ultraviolet rays.

In addition, vitamin A helps maintain healthy vision and vitamin C is well known for its role in boosting the **immune system**, so a diet that regularly includes cantaloupe melon offers many health benefits, including helping reduce the risk of cataracts and macular degeneration and helping fight infection.

Thanks to their high **potassium** content - higher even than the potassium-rich banana – cantaloupes are good for the heart. The potassium helps regulate blood pressure and eliminate 'bad' cholesterol.

✳ **storing and serving** Store ripe melons and cut melons in the refrigerator. Wrap the latter or store in an airtight container to prevent the ethylene gas they give off from affecting other fruit and vegetables.

melon with raspberries

1 Cut **2 baby cantaloupe melons** in half and scoop out and discard the seeds.

2 Spoon **125 g (4 oz) raspberries** into the hollows and top up with **300 ml (½ pint) chilled Monbazillac wine**. Chill for at least 15 minutes before serving. **serves 4**

91

NUTRITIONAL CONTENT PER 100 G: energy 17 kcals | **protein** 1 g | **carbohydrate** 3 g |

fibre 1 g | **vitamin C** 17 mg | **vitamin E** 1.2 mg | **potassium** 256 mg | **calcium** 7 mg | **magnesium** 7 mg

tomatoes

A key ingredient in the Mediterranean diet, an area famed for its low incidence of heart disease, tomatoes contain beta-carotene, vitamins C and E and **zinc**. These antioxidants help **strengthen the immune system** and reduce the risk of cataracts and other eye problems, heart disease, strokes and some cancers.

Tomatoes, the redder and riper the better, are a good source of the antioxidant lycopene, which is associated with a reduced risk of prostate and breast cancers and heart disease. Unusually for fruits and vegetables, consuming cooked or processed tomatoes, such as canned tomatoes and tomato purée, is even more beneficial than eating fresh ones.

In addition, tomatoes contain high levels of salicylates, which prevent thickening of the blood, and zinc, which is vital for fertility, especially in men. Tomatoes may help to soothe inflammation of the liver, and their high water content means they help the digestive system to function efficiently.

✴ **choosing and serving** There are numerous varieties of tomato. Sun-ripened tomatoes are the best choice, because they contain more lycopene and have a sweeter, fuller flavour than those ripened under glass. Plum tomatoes are best for cooking.

tomato and coriander salsa

1 Finely chop **1 red onion** and deseed and chop **425 g (14 oz) vine-ripened tomatoes**. Mix with **2 crushed garlic cloves** and **15 g (½ oz) chopped fresh coriander leaves**.

2 Season lightly with **salt and pepper**, cover and chill for at least 30 minutes to allow the flavours to develop.

3 Serve the salsa with cold meats or as a side dish with curries and other spicy food. **makes about 125 ml (4 fl oz)**

sweetcorn

Sweetcorn, also known as maize and corn on the cob, is a particularly good source of fibre and some B vitamins, including B_1 (thiamin), B_3 (niacin) and B_5 (pantotheic acid), which help with energy production. Vitamin B_5 is especially useful when the body is experiencing stress, while thiamin also helps preserve the memory. Another B vitamin found in high levels is **folic acid**, which helps prevent birth defects, improve the blood and protect the heart.

The fibre in sweetcorn helps **reduce high blood cholesterol levels** and protect against bowel cancer. The fibre also helps it release its energy slowly without disrupting blood sugar levels, making sweetcorn a good vegetable for diabetics.

The carotenoid zeaxanthin, which accounts for the yellow colour and is unaffected by the canning process, helps maintain healthy eyesight and protect against lung and breast cancers.

✱ **storing and serving** Choose corn with fresh-looking green husks and soft, moist silk. Warmth converts the sugar to starch, so refrigerate and eat as soon as possible. Freeze cobs and bottle the kernels.

sweetcorn cakes

1 Finely shred **4 lime leaves** and blend with **65 g (2½ oz) self-raising flour, 1 egg, 1 tablespoon Thai fish sauce, 1 tablespoon lime juice** and **75 g (3 oz) sweetcorn kernels** until fairly smooth.

2 Stir in another **75 g (3 oz) sweetcorn kernels**. Heat **5 cm (2 inches) vegetable oil** in a wok and deep-fry teaspoons of the batter, in batches, for 1–2 minutes or until golden. Drain on kitchen paper and keep warm while you cook the remainder.

3 Place a sweetcorn cake on each of **24 chicory spears**, top with a few **herb sprigs** (such as basil, mint or fresh coriander) and serve immediately. **makes about 24**

NUTRITIONAL CONTENT PER 100 G KERNELS ONLY: energy 12 kcals | protein 3 g | carbohydrates 12 g | fat 1 g | fibre 2.5 g | vitamin C 4 mg | potassium 140 mg | magnesium 20 mg

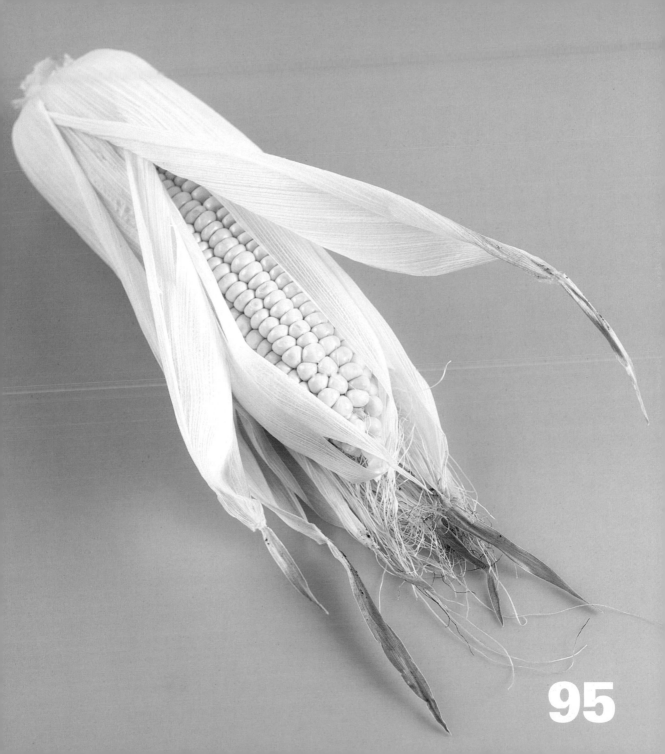

95

avocados

Nutrient-rich avocados are often shunned because of their high fat content. However, much of this fat is the monounsaturated variety and is easily digested, with none of the artery-clogging effects of saturated fat.

Avocados are **rich in the antioxidant vitamins** (A, C and E) that protect cells from the damage inflicted by free radicals and are useful for preventing conditions like heart disease. The **vitamin E** content also means that avocado helps maintain healthy skin and circulation. Not only does eating avocado provide its own antioxidants, it also improves the absorption of antioxidants from other fruit and vegetables eaten at the same time.

Avocados are good sources of the blood pressure-regulator **potassium** and the energizing B vitamins, in particular the 'anti-stress' vitamin B_5, essential for adrenal function, making them great for helping your body cope naturally with the effects of ongoing stress.

✱ storing and serving Most avocados reach the supermarket in an unripened form. As they ripen, they start to lose important antioxidant nutrients, especially vitamin C, so eat as soon as they are ripe.

avocado salsa

1 Peel, stone and finely dice **2 small ripe avocados**.

2 Finely chop **8 spring onions** and combine with the avocados, **2 tablespoons lemon juice** and **2 tablespoons chopped fresh coriander**. Season with **salt and pepper** and serve. **makes about 100 ml (3½ fl oz)**

NUTRITIONAL CONTENT PER 100 G FLESH: energy 190 kcals l **protein** 2 g l **carbohydrates** 2 g l **fat** 20 g l **fibre** 3 g l **vitamin C** 6 mg l **potassium** 450 mg l **magnesium** 25 mg

onions

Onions are a **good source of many powerful antioxidants**, which neutralize the cell-damaging free radicals in the body helping reduce the risk of strokes, heart disease, cancer, Alzheimer's disease and the other degenerative diseases of ageing. Chief among these is quercetin, which is plentiful in red onions and protects against heart disease by preventing furred arteries and blood clots from forming.

The sulphurous compounds in onions – the ones that cause tears when you slice onions – mean that a daily portion will help reduce high blood pressure and high cholesterol levels and may help protect against asthma and some inflammatory disorders, such as rheumatoid arthritis. These compounds, also found in garlic, are thought to fight cancer and **stimulate the liver's own natural detoxification process**. Indeed, research has shown that those who eat a lot of onions have lower rates of stomach cancer.

✱ storing and serving Onions can be stored for several weeks at room temperature in a dry, well-ventilated basket or vegetable rack out of direct sunlight. Keep spring onions in the refrigerator.

smooth onion soup

1 Finely chop **4 large onions** and cook gently in **3 tablespoons olive oil** for 20 minutes, stirring occasionally.

2 When the onions are soft and golden-brown, add **1.2 litres (2 pints) vegetable stock** and **2 teaspoons chopped thyme** and bring to the boil. Boil for 2 minutes, then reduce the heat, cover and simmer for 30 minutes. Add **salt and pepper** to taste.

3 Blend the soup until smooth, then return to the pan and reheat gently. Add **1 tablespoon chopped parsley** before serving. **serves 4**

NUTRITIONAL CONTENT PER 100 G: energy 36 kcals | protein 1 g | carbohydrates 8 g | fat 0 g | fibre 1.5 g | vitamin C 5 mg | potassium 160 mg | calcium 25 mg | magnesium 4 mg

broccoli

The name broccoli is applied to both white- and purple-sprouting broccoli and calabrese, the green heads sold in supermarkets. They are **powerhouses of nutrition** and should be eaten between one and three times a week for their many health-giving qualities.

All types of broccoli are rich in sulphoraphane and indoles. These stimulate the production of enzymes that help neutralize cancer-causing substances in the body and are a **major force in protecting against cancer**, particularly bowel cancer.

Broccoli also protects against heart disease and respiratory infections. It stimulates the liver, making the whole body function better, including the skin. Broccoli is a good source of **folic acid**, vital for haemoglobin formation, thus helping prevent anaemia.

Folic acid and tryptophan, an amino acid, also promote the production of the 'feel-good' neurotransmitter serotonin, so broccoli may benefit people suffering from depression and insomnia.

✱ **storing and serving** Store in the refrigerator and use within a day or so. Eat small florets raw, or boil, steam, microwave or stir-fry. Do not overcook.

broccoli sabzi

1 Stir-fry **1 teaspoon cumin seeds** in **2 tablespoons vegetable oil**. Finely slice **1 onion** and add to the pan. Cook until lightly browned.

2 Finely slice **1 red chilli** and **3 garlic cloves** and add to the pan with **300 g (10 oz) broccoli**, divided into small florets. Cover, reduce the heat and cook for 6–8 minutes, until the broccoli is just tender.

3 Season with **salt and pepper** and serve hot with a spicy curry. **serves 4**

NUTRITIONAL CONTENT PER 100 G: energy 33 kcals **| protein** 4 g **| carbohydrates** 2 g **| fat** 1 g **| fibre** 3 g **| vitamin C** 87 mg **| carotene** 535 mcg **| folate** 90 mcg **| potassium** 370 mg **| calcium** 56 mg

seaweed

Technically algae, edible seaweed is the richest food source of the mineral **iodine**, essential for normal functioning of the thyroid gland and which may help prevent breast cancer. It is also very rich in **folic acid**, which is good for preventing birth defects and linked to a reduced risk of bowel cancer.

Seaweed is great for heart health because the folic acid helps protect against heart disease and stroke, while its magnesium content helps reduce high blood pressure and heart attack. In addition, magnesium's action as a natural relaxant means that eating seaweed may help reduce the severity of asthma symptoms, prevent migraines and provide some relief from menopausal symptoms.

Including seaweed in the diet may also provide some protection from hormone-dependent cancers because the lignans (plant compounds) in seaweed have cancer-fighting properties.

Another type of algae, which is available in powdered form, **spirulina** is commonly used in juices for its energizing and health-boosting properties.

✱ **storing and serving** Increasingly available in healthfood shops and good supermarkets, seaweeds can be kept in airtight containers for several months.

seaweed and cucumber salad

1 Put **25 g (1 oz) mixed dried seaweed** (such as dulse or sea lettuce) in a bowl, cover with cold water and leave to stand for 15–20 minutes.

2 Cut **1 small cucumber** in half lengthways and slice thinly. Drain the seaweed and roughly chop any large pieces. Put the chopped seaweed in a bowl with the sliced cucumber and toss lightly. Serve as an accompaniment to grilled fish. **serves 4**

asparagus

Eat plenty of asparagus if you are trying to conceive or are in the early stages of pregnancy because it contains lots of **folic acid**, which protects against neural tube defects in the unborn baby.

The potassium-sodium balance in asparagus, combined with an amino acid called asparagine, has a **diuretic effect** so eating asparagus is good for liver and kidney function and may help alleviate bloating during menstruation.

Powerful antioxidants in asparagus – vitamins C and E and glutathione – help reduce the risk of cancer, heart disease and age-related degenerative diseases. Asparagus also contains detoxifying glucosinolates and is a source of vitamin K, which promotes blood clotting.

Avoid eating asparagus if you suffer from gout as it contains purines which increase the uric acid in the joints and exacerbate the condition.

✳ storing and serving Asparagus stalks should be straight and firm with dark, tightly furled tips. The stalk should break without bending. Keep asparagus refrigerated and try to eat on the day of purchase as flavour and vitamins quickly diminish. Serve cooked with melted butter, as Julius Caesar liked it.

hot asparagus with balsamic vinegar dressing

1 Skin, deseed and finely chop **375 g (12 oz) tomatoes** and mix with **2 tablespoons balsamic vinegar, 1–2 cloves crushed garlic** and **5 tablespoons olive oil**. Set aside.

2 Trim **500 g (1 lb) young asparagus spears**, arrange them in a single layer on a preheated, medium griddle pan and cook for 5 minutes, turning constantly.

3 Transfer the asparagus to 4 warm plates. Spoon over the dressing and top with **50 g (2 oz) toasted pine nuts** and **25 g (1 oz) Parmesan shavings**. Season and serve at once. **serves 4**

NUTRITIONAL CONTENT PER 100 G: energy 25 kcals | **protein** 3 g | **carbohydrates** 2 g | **fat** 1 g | **fibre** 2 g | **vitamin C** 12 mg | **folate** 175 mcg | **potassium** 260 mg | **calcium** 27 mg

105

peas

Fresh peas are one of the richest fresh vegetable sources of **iron** and also contain a good amount of vitamin B₁ (thiamin). The iron can help prevent anaemia, while the thiamin is required to convert food into energy and help maintain a healthy heart and nervous system.

The soluble fibre in peas makes them a **good choice for diabetics** because it both slows down the release of energy and stabilizes blood sugar levels. The fibre also helps protect the heart by reducing cholesterol levels.

The green pigment in peas, chlorophyllin, can help prevent cancer because it carries free radicals out of the body. Plant hormones, lignans, are thought to protect against hormone-dependent cancers as well as menopausal problems.

The carotenoids lutein and zaethanin help maintain healthy eyes, and **folic acid** can help prevent birth defects and helping reduce the risk of heart disease.

✱ **storing and serving** Fresh peas need to be kept in the refrigerator to preserve their texture, flavour and nutrients. They are best eaten on the day of purchase. Frozen peas are as good, or better, a source as fresh ones for vitamin C.

summer green pea soup

1 Trim, wash and chop a **bunch of spring onions** and soften in **15 g (½ oz) butter**. Do not allow them to colour.

2 Shell **1.25 kg (2½ lb) fresh peas** (or use 500 g (1 lb) frozen peas) and add them to the pan with **750 ml (1¼ pints) vegetable stock**. Bring to the boil and simmer for about 15 minutes (5 minutes for frozen peas).

3 Blend the soup until smooth and return to the pan. Stir in **2 tablespoons natural yogurt**, reheat gently and serve, sprinkled with **1 tablespoon chopped chives**. serves 4

green beans

The term green beans covers all types of thick or skinny, long, fresh beans with small seeds inside.

Eating green beans **helps maintain bone strength** because they are a great source of vitamin K. They also contain many nutrients with heart-protective qualities, including the antioxidant vitamins A and C, which **neutralize damaging free radicals** and help prevent clogged arteries; potassium and magnesium, which work together to **lower high blood pressure**; folic acid, which protects against heart attack and stroke by preventing the harmful build-up of the amino acid homocysteine; and soluble fibre, which helps **lower blood cholesterol**.

The fibre in beans helps keep the digestive system healthy and prevent bowel cancer by removing toxins from the body. Richer in **iron** than spinach, green beans can help prevent fatigue and anaemia.

✱ **storing and serving** Green beans keep in the refrigerator for a few days. Blanch and use in salads or with dips, or steam or stir-fry them. Canned and frozen beans retain about half their original vitamin C content.

green bean and tomato salad

1 Halve **250 g (8 oz) red and yellow baby plum tomatoes** and put them in a large bowl.

2 Trim **250 g (8 oz) thin green beans**, cook for 2 minutes, drain well and add to the tomatoes.

3 Add a **handful of chopped mint**, **1 crushed garlic clove**, **4 tablespoons olive oil** and **1 tablespoon balsamic vinegar**. Season with **salt and pepper** and mix well. Serve warm or cold. **serves 4**

NUTRITIONAL CONTENT PER 100 G: energy 24 kcals | **protein** 2 g | **carbohydrates** 3 g | **fat** 1 g | **fibre** 3 g | **vitamin C** 12 mg | **folate** 80 mcg | **potassium** 230 mg | **calcium** 36 mg | **iron** 1.2 mg

109

broad beans

Archaeological evidence suggests that broad beans, also known as fava (faba), horse and Windsor beans, were cultivated in Neolithic times, making them one of the first crops to be cultivated.

A good source of protein, they are ideal for vegetarians. The fibre they contain helps keep the digestive system healthy, so helps **protect against bowel cancer** and **lower blood cholesterol levels**.

Broad beans are a good choice for women in the early stages of pregnancy as they contain **folic acid**. And they are good for controlling blood pressure as their **potassium** helps regulate fluid levels in the body.

Broad beans are known to provoke a severe allergic reaction called favism in a small group of people of Mediterranean or Middle Eastern origin – where the bean originated.

✻ storing and serving To avoid flavour loss, keep broad beans in the refrigerator and use as soon as possible. The pods of young broad beans are edible.

broad bean and pecorino salad

1 Shell **375 g (12 oz) fresh broad beans** and blanch in boiling water for 2 minutes. Drain and refresh. If you have time, after blanching the beans, remove the outer skins to reveal the bright green, velvety bean inside.

2 Coarsely grate **175 g (6 oz) pecorino cheese** and put it in a mixing bowl. Add the beans, **2 tablespoons each of olive oil** and **lemon juice** and **1 tablespoon chopped flat-leaf parsley**. Season with **salt and pepper** and mix well. Serve as part of an antipasto. **serves 4**

NUTRITIONAL CONTENT PER 100 G: energy 59 kcals I **protein** 6 g I **carbohydrates** 7 g I **fat** 1 g I **fibre** 6 g I **vitamin C** 32 mg I **folate** 145 mcg I **potassium** 310 mg I **calcium** 23 mg

mangetout

Mangetout, also known as snow peas, are flat, wide, edible pods with little bulges indicating the small, immature peas. Their nutritional profile is similar to that of garden peas, although the immature seeds account for some differences – there is less protein in mangetout, for example. However, they provide twice the **calcium** and slightly more **iron** than garden peas and are a better source of beta-carotene (vitamin A).

The iron and **folic acid** in mangetout means they can help build red blood cells and so are good for people susceptible to anaemia. Folic acid can also help prevent birth defects. In addition, it may help keep heart and blood vessels healthy.

The fibre in mangetouts also helps prevent cancer by keeping the digestive system working efficiently, and it can protect the heart by **reducing blood cholesterol levels**.

✱ storing and serving Keep mangetout in the refrigerator and use as soon as possible after purchase. Eat them raw or only slightly cooked so as to retain some 'crunch' as well as their nutrients; they are ideal in stir-fries or they can be steamed. Rinse before cooking and 'top and tail' the pods.

mangetout with ginger and mint

1 Cut **5 cm (2 inch) fresh root ginger** into matchsticks and stir-fry in **2 tablespoons olive oil** for 1–2 minutes to flavour the oil.

2 Trim **500 g (1 lb) mangetout**, add to the pan and stir-fry for 2 minutes.

3 Remove from the heat and stir **2 teaspoons lemon juice** and **2 tablespoons chopped mint**. Season to taste with **salt and pepper** and serve at once, garnished with **mint sprigs**. serves 4–6

NUTRITIONAL CONTENT PER 100 G RAW: energy 32 kcals | **protein** 4 g | **carbohydrates** 4 g | **fat** 0 g | **fibre** 4 g | **vitamin C** 21 mg | **potassium** 200 mg | **calcium** 44 mg | **iron** 0.8 mg

113

okra

Also known as bhindi and lady's fingers, okra is a member of the cotton family and originated in Africa. It is a green (sometimes white), tapering seed capsule, which has its own unique flavour and texture.

Okra is high in dietary fibre, which helps keep the digestive system healthy and protects the heart by **lowering high blood cholesterol levels**. Okra contains even more **potassium** than bananas and this can help regulate fluid levels in the body and is therefore important for controlling blood pressure.

Okra is also a good source of vitamin C – essential for boosting immunity and for general good health – and a number of B vitamins, including **folic acid**. Taken by mothers-to-be, folic acid can help protect babies from neural tube defects. It also boosts red blood cells, helping to combat fatigue and anaemia.

✱ storing and serving Choose small, young pods that have not yet matured and toughened. Once cut, okra oozes a slimy sap, which is ideal for thickening soups and stews but is not to everyone's taste. To minimize this sap, cut okra only just before cooking and cook it quickly.

bhindi bhaji

1 Heat **3 tablespoons vegetable oil** and add **1 tablespoon mustard seeds** and **1 tablespoon cumin seeds**.

2 Trim **500 g (1 lb) okra** and cut into 1 cm (½ inch) slices. When the mustard seeds begin to pop, add the okra and stir-fry for 8–10 minutes.

3 Add **1 teaspoon chilli powder**, **1 tablespoon dhana-jeera**, **2 teaspoons jaggery** (or soft brown sugar) and **1 finely chopped tomato** and cook for 3–5 minutes. Remove from the heat, season with **salt and pepper** and stir in **2 tablespoons chopped fresh coriander**. Serve hot with **lime wedges**, if liked. **serves 4**

NUTRITIONAL CONTENT PER 100 G RAW: energy 31 kcals | **protein** 3 g | **carbohydrates** 3 g | **fat** 1 g | **fibre** 5 g | **vitamin C** 21 mg | **folate** 88 mcg | **potassium** 330 mg | **calcium** 160 mg

peppers

Red, yellow and orange peppers are simply riper versions of green ones, and their longer maturing time increases their overall nutrient content.

All peppers, especially red ones, contain high levels of the antioxidants vitamin C, beta-carotene (vitamin A), **vitamin E** and **zinc**, so they fight off free radicals and protect against heart disease, strokes and some cancers. These same nutrients are vital for a **strong immune system** and for energy production.

Vitamin C and the magnesium in peppers work together to produce adrenaline, which makes peppers great for helping the body deal with stress.

Red peppers contain the red carotenoid lycopene, which helps prevent prostate cancer, and lutein and zeaxanthin, which both protect against vision problems such as cataracts and macular degeneration.

Other chemicals in peppers help prevent constipation, especially if drunk in fresh juice or eaten raw.

✱ **storing and serving** Choose firm, unwrinkled peppers and store in the refrigerator. All colours can be eaten raw or cooked and can even be juiced.

roasted stuffed peppers

1 Halve, core and deseed **4 large red peppers**. Put the peppers, cut sides up, in a ceramic dish. Scatter over **2 crushed garlic cloves** and **1 tablespoon chopped thyme** and season with **salt and pepper**.

2 Halve **4 plum tomatoes** and put a piece in each pepper. Drizzle with a mixture of **4 tablespoons olive oil** and **2 tablespoons balsamic vinegar** and roast in a preheated oven, 220°C (425°F), Gas Mark 7, for 55–60 minutes or until the peppers are soft and charred. Serve with crusty bread and a baby leaf salad. **serves 4**

NUTRITIONAL CONTENT PER 100 G RED RAW: energy 32 kcals | **protein** 1 g | **carbohydrates** 6 g | **fat** 0 g | **fibre** 2 g | **vitamin C** 140 mg | **carotene** 3840 mcg | **potassium** 160 mg

117

carrots

Carrots are probably the richest vegetable source of carotenoids. These antioxidants and the other nutrients in carrots – fibre, **calcium**, **potassium**, magnesium, vitamins C and E, among others – give the vegetable plenty of health-boosting powers.

Carrots are vital for the **immune system** and protect against heart and arterial diseases and cancer. They also help regulate blood sugar levels and **reduce blood cholesterol** levels, and they are vital for building strong teeth, hair and bones. Easy to digest and good for internal cleansing, carrots have beneficial effects on the digestive system and skin as well as on the respiratory system.

The beta-carotene in carrots is also believed to promote good eyesight, especially night vision. In addition, beta-carotene, lutein and zeaxanthin help to **protect the eyes** from ultraviolet light and reduce the risk of cataracts and macular degeneration.

✱ storing and serving Store carrots in a plastic bag in the refrigerator, first removing their green tops if they are still attached to prevent them drying out. Scrub carrots well and, unless they are organic, peel them to avoid ingesting pesticide residues. Juicing is a popular way to benefit from the goodness in carrots.

carrot and coriander pâté

1 Grate **500 g (1 lb) carrots** and put them in a saucepan with **1 tablespoon ground coriander, 175 ml (6 fl oz) orange juice** and **300 ml (½ pint) water.** Cover and simmer for 40 minutes or until the carrots are cooked. Leave to cool.

2 Drain quickly and transfer to food processor with a little of the cooking liquid. Add **50 g (2 oz) medium-fat soft cheese** and **30 g (1¼ oz) fresh coriander.** Blend until smooth, season with **salt and pepper** and blend again.

3 Chill and serve with country bread or toast. **serves 4**

fennel

Florence fennel, the swollen, bulb-like leaf base of a relative of the herb fennel, contains **phyto-oestrogens**, compounds produced naturally in plants that mimic the female hormone oestrogen. Women may therefore find fennel useful for dealing with premenstrual syndrome (PMS) and for relieving some menopausal symptoms, such as hot flushes. Phyto-oestrogens are also thought to offer some protection against hormone-related cancers.

Fennel contains a good range of antioxidants, including two flavonoids, quercetin and rutin, and vitamin C, which means that fennel has **anti-cancer** and **anti-microbial** properties and that it provides a good boost to the **immune system**.

The **potassium** and fibre in fennel are great for the health of the heart and digestive system. Fibre also helps reduce the risk of bowel cancer.

✱ storing and serving Florence fennel has a distinctive aniseed flavour. It may be eaten raw in salads, or cooked, usually by braising, steaming or baking. The leaves and seeds of the herbaceous perennial fennel are used as herbs and seasonings. Fennel tea is a useful digestive aid after a rich meal.

braised fennel with pecorino

1 Melt **50 g (2 oz) butter** in a large pan. When it stops foaming, add **12 baby fennel bulbs**, trimmed and halved lengthways, and fry gently for 2 minutes on each side until lightly golden. Add **150 ml (¼ pint) water** and a **squeeze of lemon juice**. Season with **salt and pepper**, bring to the boil, cover and simmer for 20 minutes or until the fennel is tender.

2 Add **1 tablespoon balsamic vinegar** and increase the heat to reduce the liquid by half. Remove the pan from the heat, add **3–4 tablespoons grated pecorino cheese** and allow the cheese to melt. Serve the fennel and pan juices with new potatoes. **serves 4**

NUTRITIONAL CONTENT PER 100 G RAW: energy 12 kcals I protein 1 g I carbohydrates 2 g I fat 0 g I fibre 2 g I vitamin C 5 mg I potassium 440 mg I calcium 24 mg I magnesium 8 mg

121

spinach

Spinach is an important source of the antioxidants beta-carotene and vitamins C and E, which strengthen the **immune system** and reduce the risk of heart disease and stroke as well as some cancers. The carotenoids in spinach may also protect against cataracts and macular degeneration.

Although spinach is best known for its **high iron content**, these levels are not as high as once thought. Iron helps prevent fatigue and anaemia.

The vitamin K and magnesium in spinach help **build healthy blood cells**, while the **calcium** builds bones and teeth and helps prevent osteoarthritis.

Spinach is a good source of **folic acid**, which builds up red blood cells and is essential in early pregnancy for helping to protect babies from spina bifida.

Spinach is also a natural laxative but the oxalic acid in the leaves makes it unsuitable for people with kidney or bladder stones.

✱ **storing and serving** Spinach may be stored in a bag in the refrigerator for a few days. Wash the leaves then shake dry for use in a salad. Alternatively, steam quickly using just the water clinging to the leaves.

bacon, spinach and blue cheese salad

1 Chop **3 rashers of rindless smoked back bacon** and fry until crisp. Add **25 g (1 oz) pine nuts** and cook for 1–2 minutes until the nuts begin to brown.

2 Wash **225 g (7½ oz) fresh baby spinach**, dice **50 g (2 oz) Gorgonzola cheese** and halve **12 cherry tomatoes** and stir into the bacon and pine nuts. Transfer the salad to a serving bowl.

3 Mix together **1 teaspoon wholegrain mustard, 1 teaspoon clear honey** and **2 tablespoons balsamic vinegar**. Pour the dressing over the salad and serve with crusty bread. **serves 4**

NUTRITIONAL CONTENT PER 100 G FRESH, RAW: energy 25 kcals | **protein** 3 g | **carbohydrates** 2 g | **fat** 1 g | **fibre** 4 g | **vitamin C** 26 mg | **carotene** 3535 mcg | **vitamin E** 1.7 mg

mushrooms

Classed as a fungus rather than a vegetable, mushrooms are an excellent source of **selenium**, an **anti-cancer** mineral that can limit the damage inflicted in the body by free radicals. Mushrooms are believed to offer protection against breast cancer thanks to their part in regulating levels of oestrogen in the body.

Fresh and dried mushrooms are rich in phytochemicals that protect the body when it is under stress, particularly vitamin B_5, which is essential for adrenal function and improves the body's coping mechanisms.

The **potassium** present in mushrooms helps regulate the body's fluid levels, including blood pressure.

Research has shown **oriental mushrooms** to be more health-boosting than common mushrooms. They are thought to help prevent blood clots. Shiitake and reishi mushrooms contain the phytochemical lentinan, believed to prevent and treat cancer and viral diseases as well as **reducing high blood cholesterol levels** and high blood pressure.

✱ **storing and serving** Keep button mushrooms in the refrigerator in a paper bag for 1–2 days. Use field mushrooms as soon as possible after purchase.

roast mushrooms on toast

1 Put **8 large mushrooms**, in a roasting tin and season with **salt and pepper**. In a bowl mix together **2 crushed garlic cloves**, **125 ml (4 fl oz) olive oil**, **2 teaspoons chopped thyme** and the finely grated rind of **1 lemon**. Spoon half of the sauce over the mushrooms.

2 Roast the mushrooms in a preheated oven, 220°C (425°F), Gas Mark 7, for 20 minutes. Drizzle over **4 tablespoons lemon juice**.

3 Put the mushrooms on 4 slices of **buttered toast**, drizzle over the remaining sauce and serve topped with **rocket leaves** and shavings of **Parmesan cheese**. **serves 4**

NUTRITIONAL CONTENT PER 100 G RAW: energy 13 kcals | **protein** 2 g | **carbohydrates** 0 g | **fat** 1 g | **fibre** 2 g | **vitamin C** 1 mg | **potassium** 320 mg | **calcium** 6 mg | **selenium** 9 mcg

126

yams

In the USA the word yam is sometimes applied to sweet potatoes with yellow flesh, and yams are often confused with sweet potatoes, but they are different, unrelated vegetables. The hundreds of varieties account for yams' varying flesh and skin colours, which only add to the confusion. They are usually long and cylindrical, however, with rough, scaly skin.

The antioxidants **vitamin C** and **manganese** in yams provide protection against free radicals. Yams also contain lots of **potassium** (even more than bananas) and vitamin B$_6$, two nutrients that help protect the heart. Potassium helps regulate blood pressure, so it is useful for dealing with hypertension, while vitamin B$_6$ breaks down homocysteine, a substance that can damage blood vessel walls resulting in strokes and heart attacks.

A good energizing food, yams release their carbohydrates slowly into the body, helping stabilize blood sugar levels.

✱ **storing and serving** Toxic if eaten raw but perfectly safe when cooked, yams can generally be substituted in recipes that call for sweet potato. Their tough skins are easier to remove after cooking, but wash and peel before mashing or roasting.

yam mash

1 Peel and roughly chop **750 g (1½ lb) yams**. Cook in boiling water for 20–30 minutes or until soft.

2 Meanwhile, briefly dry-fry then roughly crush **1 teaspoon each of cumin seeds and coriander seeds**.

3 Drain the yams and mash with the crushed cumin and coriander, **3 tablespoons olive oil** and **4 tablespoons natural yogurt (or crème fraîche)**. Season with **salt and pepper**, then serve. serves 4

sweet potatoes

The sweet potato is a different species from the yam, with which it is often confused. Sweet potatoes are **packed with carotenoids**, including the vision-protecting lutein, and zeaxanthin as well as beta-carotene (vitamin A) and vitamin C, which both have antioxidant and **anti-inflammatory** properties. Sweet potatoes are therefore good for fighting the free radicals responsible for clogged arteries, heart disease, stroke, cancer and age-related eye diseases. They help reduce inflammation in asthma and rheumatoid arthritis.

Another antioxidant in sweet potatoes is **vitamin E**, which is good for the skin and can soothe skin conditions such as eczema.

Loaded with starchy carbohydrates and fibre, sweet potatoes release their sugars slowly into the bloodstream, providing long-lasting energy, and can help stabilize blood sugar levels.

✱ storing and serving Store sweet potatoes for several days in a cool, dark, airy place. Do not keep them in the refrigerator. Eat the skins if they are organic. Bake, steam, boil or roast them.

baked sweet potatoes with salsa

1 Scrub **2 sweet potatoes**, each about 275 g (9 oz), and put them in a roasting tin. Prick with a fork and drizzle with **1 tablespoon olive oil** and a little **salt**. Bake in a preheated oven, 200°C (400°F), Gas Mark 6, for 45 minutes.

2 Chop **2 large tomatoes**, ½ **small red onion** and **1 celery stick** and mix with a **small handful of chopped fresh coriander**, **2 tablespoons lime juice** and **2 teaspoons caster sugar**.

3 Halve the sweet potatoes and sprinkle with **50 g (2 oz) grated Emmental cheese** and serve topped with the salsa. **serves 2**

NUTRITIONAL CONTENT PER 100 G RAW, YELLOW FLESH: energy 87 kcals | **protein** 1 g | **carbohydrates** 21 g | **fat** 0 g | **fibre** 2 g | **vitamin C** 23 mg | **carotene** 3930 mcg | **vitamin E** 4.56 mg

129

pumpkins and butternut squashes

Sharing a similar flavour and texture, pumpkins and butternut squashes are different types of winter squash. Their superb carotenoid content includes lutein and zeaxanthin, which **help protect vision**; and beta-cryptoxanthin, which has been shown to protect against lung and prostate cancers and improve joint health.

Beta-carotene has powerful antioxidant and **anti-inflammatory** properties, so eating pumpkins and butternut squashes can help prevent the clogged arteries that lead to strokes and heart attacks. It may also help reduce the risk of bowel cancer and alleviate inflammatory conditions, such as rheumatoid arthritis.

Both pumpkins and butternut squashes have plenty of fibre, which helps the digestive system function smoothly, especially in people suffering from **irritable bowel syndrome (IBS)**.

✱ **storing and serving** Uncut winter squashes will keep well in a cool, dry place for several months. Use them in sweet and savoury dishes. Bake or roast them for use in hearty stews, or purée for soups.

roasted pumpkin with walnut and rocket pesto

1 Cut a **1 kg (2 lb) pumpkin** into 8 wedges and discard the seeds. Brush with **olive oil**, season with **salt and pepper** and roast in a preheated oven, 220°C (425°F), Gas Mark 7, for 20–25 minutes, turning halfway through.

2 Trim and chop **2 spring onions** and crush **1 large garlic clove**. Blend with **50 g (2 oz) toasted walnuts** and **50 g (2 oz) rocket leaves** until finely chopped. Blend in **3 tablespoons walnut oil** and **3 tablespoons olive oil**. Season with **salt and pepper**. **serves 4**

NUTRITIONAL CONTENT PER 100 G RAW PUMPKIN (BUTTERNUT): energy 13 (36) kcals | **protein** 1 (1) g | **carbohydrates** 2 (8) g | **fat** 0 (0) g | **fibre** 1 (2) g | **carotene** 450 (3630) mcg

131

NUTRITIONAL CONTENT PER 100 G RAW: energy 26 kcals | **protein** 2 g | **carbohydrates** 4 g | **fat** 0 g | **fibre** 3 g | **vitamin C** 49 mg | **carotene** 385 mcg | **vitamin E** 0.2 mg | **potassium** 270 mg

cabbage

All types of cabbage (red, green and white) are highly nutritious and rich in cancer-fighting glucosinolates – green cabbage has especially high levels. These phytochemicals, including sulphoraphane and indoles, **inhibit the growth of tumours** and appear to protect against bowel, ovarian and breast cancers.

Raw cabbage is great for detoxifying the digestive system, soothing indigestion and the after-effects of stomach upsets, and helps treat constipation.

Cabbage contains high levels of the antioxidant vitamins A, C and E, so it helps protect against free-radical damage. The vitamin C content helps to build up resistance to coughs, colds and other infections.

Pak choi (bok choy) and Savoy cabbage are richer in nutrients than other green and white cabbages. Red cabbage contains the most antioxidants. The vivid colour is due to anthocyanidins, potent antioxidants with **anti-cancer**, **anti-microbial** and **anti-inflammatory** properties.

✱ **storing and serving** Store whole cabbages in a cool, dry place for several days. Once cut, cover the surface tightly with clingfilm, keep in the refrigerator and use within a day or so. Use cabbage raw in juices or salads. Steam or stir-fry to retain more nutrients.

stir-fried Chinese cabbage

1 Cut **8–10 large Chinese cabbage leaves** diagonally into thin strips.

2 Drain and slice **125 g (4 oz) canned bamboo shoots**, slice **1 onion** and **1 celery stick** and fry gently in **2 tablespoons vegetable oil** for about 8 minutes, stirring frequently.

3 Add a little **lemon juice** and season with **salt and pepper** to taste. Serve garnished with **lemon slices. serves 4**

watercress

The distinctive, peppery taste of watercress has made it a popular garnish, but you should use it for more than livening up a dull salad to make the most of its health-boosting properties. Watercress is a **powerful detoxifier** and contains the antioxidants beta-carotene (vitamin A) and vitamins C and E and **zinc**. These fortify the **immune system** and reduce the risk of heart disease, strokes and some cancers.

Watercress contains beneficial isothiocyanates, which protect against a known tobacco-borne carcinogen and therefore help reduce the risk of lung cancer in smokers.

Eating watercress can help to **reduce blood cholesterol** levels, and its high **iron** content prevents or reduces anaemia.

Watercress is an appetite stimulant so is useful for people with small appetites after illness. It is also mildly diuretic and laxative. It can help dissolve kidney and bladder stones.

✱ **storing and serving** Watercress is best eaten on the day of purchase. Cut away the coarse stems and use the leaves in salads, sandwiches and soups.

chilled watercress and pear soup

1 Coarsley chop **2 bunches watercress** and cook in **50 g (2 oz) butter** for 3 minutes, stirring frequently. Peel, core and slice **3 pears** and add to the pan with **1 litre (1¾ pints) vegetable stock**, a **pinch of grated nutmeg** and **pepper** to taste.

2 Bring to the boil then reduce the heat, cover and simmer for 15–20 minutes. Process to a smooth purée when cool. Stir in **2 tablespoons lemon juice**, cover tightly with clingfilm and refrigerate for at least 3 hours.

3 Fold in **150 ml (¼ pint) single cream** and serve. **serves 4–6**

NUTRITIONAL CONTENT PER 100 G: energy 22 kcals | **protein** 3 g | **carbohydrates** 0 g | **fat** 1 g | **fibre** 3 g | **vitamin C** 62 mg | **carotene** 2520 mcg | **vitamin E** 1.46 mg | **iron** 2.2 mg | **zinc** 0.7 mg

136

radishes

Radishes are believed to have been cultivated in Egypt before 2000 BC, and from there they spread to China and Japan. Of the many different varieties of radish, the best known are probably the small red, white-fleshed globes. There are, however, many other colours and shapes, including the longer-rooted types available in winter. Skin colours include yellow and black as well as red, and there are even radishes with red flesh.

Radishes are related to the brassicas (a family that includes cabbage, kale and broccoli) and contain significant quantities of the same sulphurous compounds. By **inhibiting the production of cancerous cells**, these glucosinolates are a major force in protecting against cancer.

The same phytochemicals are good for the digestive system and help relieve indigestion and flatulence. Radishes are great for boosting the **immune system**.

The daikon, or mooli, is an oriental radish with a long white root, often juiced for its properties as a blood cleanser and appetite stimulant.

✳ storing and serving Radishes will keep in the refrigerator for a day or two. Common radishes are usually eaten raw. Oriental radishes may also be eaten raw but are more often included in stir-fries or pickles.

fresh ricotta with herb oil and radishes

1 Cut **375 g (12 oz) ricotta cheese** into thin wedges and arrange them on a plate. Combine **50 ml (2 fl oz) olive oil** and **1 tablespoon chopped herbs** (such as basil, chives, mint or parsley), season with **salt and pepper** and drizzle over the ricotta.

2 Wash and trim a **bunch of radishes** and arrange around the edge of the plate. Serve with crusty bread. **serves 4**

lettuce

In ancient Egypt lettuce was sacred to Min, the god of male fertility, but now herbal remedies containing lettuce are **recommended for insomnia**.

Although lettuces consist of 95 per cent water, they are still nutritious. The darker the leaves, the more nutrients they contain, and for this reason cos (or romaine) and red-leaved lettuces are far more health-boosting than the pale iceberg types. The darker lettuces are great for eye health thanks to the antioxidant carotenoids lutein and zeaxanthin, which filter the high-energy light waves responsible for free-radical damage to the eyes. They may, therefore, help reduce the risk of age-related macular degeneration.

Like all leafy greens, lettuce is an important food for women trying to conceive or in the early stages of pregnancy thanks to its **folic acid**.

✱ **storing and serving** Uniquely among vegetables, lettuces are available only in their fresh state. Store them in the refrigerator and eat as soon as possible after purchase. Firm lettuces, such as cos (romaine) and iceberg, will last longer than soft-leaved lettuces. Lettuces can be braised or included in soups.

smoked chicken and avocado salad

1 Cut **500 g (1 lb) smoked chicken breast** into bite-size pieces and place them in a large bowl. Add the leaves from **3 cos lettuce hearts**. Peel, stone and slice **1 large ripe avocado** and add to the bowl with **25 g (1 oz) grated Parmesan cheese**. Toss well and serve at once. **serves 4**

NUTRITIONAL CONTENT PER 100 G COS: energy 16 kcals | **protein** 1 g | **carbohydrates** 2 g | **fat** 1 g | **fibre** 1 g | **vitamin C** 5 mg | **carotene** 290 mcg | **folate** 55 mcg | **potassium** 220 mg

139

NUTRITIONAL CONTENT PER 100 G RAW: energy 33 kcals | protein 3 g | carbohydrates 1 g | fat 2 g | fibre 3 g | vitamin C 110 mg | carotene 3145 mcg | vitamin E 1.7 mg | calcium 130 mg

kale

A leafy green vegetable from the brassica family, kale is possibly the closest modern vegetable to a wild cabbage, but the thick-stemmed leaves do not form a head. Kale has the same **cancer-protective sulphurous phytochemicals** as cabbage. These stimulate the body to produce cancer-fighting enzymes and inhibit tumour growth, and they also appear to protect against bowel, ovarian and breast cancers.

Kale is a really good source of the antioxidant vitamins A, C and E, which protect against heart disease and cancer and **strengthen the immune system**. Lutein and zeaxanthin are two carotenoids found in kale, which **protect the eyes** from ultraviolet light and help prevent problems like cataracts.

Perhaps surprisingly, kale has more available **calcium** than cow's milk. Calcium is essential for healthy bones, so kale is a good choice for those who want the calcium without the calories or who are allergic to dairy products.

✶ storing and serving Store kale in the refrigerator and use it quickly as it becomes more bitter as time passes. Kale is usually steamed or stir-fried, although young leaves can be used raw in salads and in juices.

colcannon

1 Shred and remove the stalks of **500 g (1 lb) kale** and cook for 10 minutes. Boil **500 g (1 lb) unpeeled potatoes** in another pan until tender.

2 Meanwhile, finely chop **6 spring onions** and gently simmer in **150 ml (¼ pint) milk** for 5 minutes.

3 Drain, peel and mash the potatoes. Add the hot milk and beat well. Drain the kale and beat into the potato with **50 g (2 oz) butter**. Season with **salt and pepper**. Heat through and serve with extra butter. **serves 4–6**

beetroot

Beetroot is closely related to mangelwurzels and sugar beet. It contains high levels of beta-carotene and vitamin C, which help fight off infection and diseases.

Beetroot also contains **vitamin B$_6$**, **folic acid**, **calcium**, **iron**, manganese, magnesium, phosphorus and potassium, which help improve the functioning of the kidneys, gall bladder and liver and help the body to develop healthy bones, teeth and muscles. Don't eat too much beetroot if you have kidney stones, however, as the high levels of oxalates in the vegetable block the body's absorption of **calcium** and iron.

The iron and folic acid in beetroot help build up red blood cells, **preventing fatigue and anaemia**. Folic acid also has a role in preventing heart disease and cancer. The iron and manganese in beetroot help to alleviate particularly low haemoglobin levels caused by very heavy periods, and menopausal problems.

✱ storing and serving Raw, freshly cooked and canned beetroot contain more nutrients than pickled beetroot. Beetroot can also be used in soups, notably the Russian and Polish favourite borsch.

beetroot and sugar snap pasta

1 Cook **250 g (8 oz) pasta** according to the instructions on the packet.

2 Meanwhile, peel and chop **250 g (8 oz) cooked beetroot**. Trim **125 g (4 oz) sugar snap peas**, cut them into thirds and blanch in boiling water for 1 minute.

3 Drain the pasta, return it to the pan and add the beetroot and peas. Stir over a low heat for 2 minutes.

4 Remove from the heat. and stir in **200 ml (7 fl oz) crème fraîche**, **2 tablespoons chopped fresh chives, salt and pepper**. Serve topped with **grated Parmesan cheese. serves 4**

NUTRITIONAL CONTENT PER 100 G RAW: energy 36 kcals | protein 2 g | carbohydrates 8 g | fat 0 g | fibre 3 g | vitamin C 5 mg | potassium 380 mg | calcium 20 mg | magnesium 11 mg

potatoes

A source of filling starchy carbohydrates, potatoes are a great energizing and low-fat food. Eating endless supplies of potato crisps and chips, however, will not give you the benefit of their health-boosting properties!

Potatoes are a good source of **potassium**, which helps reduce high blood pressure. The fibre, especially in the skins, is great for **reducing blood cholesterol levels** and maintaining a healthy digestive system. They also contain vitamin C, which **boosts the immune system**, and cell-building vitamin B_6.

Anyone suffering from depression should eat plenty of potatoes as they are thought to boost production of the brain chemical serotonin, which helps improve mood.

Potatoes may also reduce the risk of bowel and liver cancers thanks to a phytonutrient called chlorogenic acid, which may inhibit the formation of some carcinogens.

✱ storing and serving Some types of potato are better than others for the different methods of cooking. Pre-packaged potatoes often indicate the best cooking method on the bag. Store potatoes in a cool, dark, airy place but not in the refrigerator. Leave them unpeeled if possible to benefit from the most nutrients.

roasted paprika potato wedges

1 Scrub **4 baking potatoes**, each about 250 g (8 oz) each, and cut each lengthways into 8 wedges.

2 Place in a roasting tin, drizzle with **4 tablespoons olive oil** and toss well to coat. Sprinkle with **1–2 teaspoons paprika** and season with **salt**.

3 Cook in a preheated oven, 220°C (425°F), Gas Mark 7, for 35–40 minutes, basting with the oil 2–3 times during cooking, until the wedges are tender and nicely browned.

4 Serve as a side dish or as a starter with soured cream, aïoli or mayonnaise. **serves 4**

NUTRITIONAL CONTENT PER 100 G, WHOLE BAKED: energy 136 kcals | **protein** 4 g | **carbohydrates** 32 g | **fat** 0.2 g | **fibre** 3 g | **vitamin C** 14 mg | **vitamin B_6** 0.54 mg | **potassium** 630 mg

145

cauliflowers

Some sources say cauliflowers originated in China and were introduced into Spain in the 12th century. Others say they were an east Mediterranean crop, exported to Italy as recently as the late 15th century. Originally, the heads were no larger than tennis balls, but plants with huge heads gradually became popular.

Like other vegetables in the brassica family with the same **cancer-inhibiting sulphurous compounds**, cauliflower has an important role in fighting cancer, especially hormonal, bowel and lung cancers.

The fibre in cauliflower makes it a heart-protective vegetable because it helps **lower blood cholesterol** levels, and the **folic acid** helps neutralize excessive levels of heart attack-causing homocysteine.

Cauliflower is a good choice for women before or during early pregnancy because folic acid can help prevent birth defects, and its vitamin C content is good for **strengthening the immune system**.

✱ storing and serving Keep cauliflowers in the refrigerator and use within 1–2 days. Florets can be eaten raw in salads. The briefer the cooking time for cauliflower, the less smelly the sulphurous compounds.

cauliflower relish

1 Cook **2 teaspoons black mustard seeds**, **½ teaspoon each of ground turmeric** and **asafoetida** in **2 tablespoons vegetable oil**.

2 Cut **1 small cauliflower** into bite-size pieces, finely chop **1 red onion** and deseed and chop **1 fresh green chilli**. When the seeds start to pop, add the vegetables and stir-fry for 5 minutes. The cauliflower should be firm to bite.

3 Season to taste with **lemon juice** and **salt** and serve at room temperature. **serves 4**

NUTRITIONAL CONTENT PER 100 G RAW: energy 34 kcals | **protein** 4 g | **carbohydrates** 3 g | **fat** 1 g | **fibre** 2 g | **vitamin C** 43 mg | **folate** 66 mcg | **potassium** 380 mg | **calcium** 21 mg

147

148

globe artichokes

The edible bud of a type of thistle, globe artichokes may be fiddly to eat but are worth the effort. According to researchers at the US Department of Agriculture (USDA), they are the **best vegetable source of antioxidants** – even better than broccoli and spinach.

Globe artichokes have detoxifying qualities and help the liver eliminate toxins from the body more effectively, which helps improve the skin. A phytonutrient called cynarine stimulates the liver's production of bile, which aids digestion and may even help alleviate irritable bowel syndrome (IBS). They are good for heart health, too, as cynarine can also help **lower blood cholesterol** levels and reduce blood pressure.

The **folic acid** in globe artichokes makes them a good choice for pregnant women or those trying to conceive.

✱ **storing and serving** Fresh globe artichokes will keep for only a few days in the refrigerator. Remove the inedible tips of the leaves and twist off the stalk before cooking and serving with butter or mayonnaise. Ready-to-eat artichoke hearts are available frozen or in cans or jars. Serve these as antipasti or in salads or stir-fries.

artichoke and dill soup

1 Chop **1 onion** and **1 garlic clove** and slice **1 celery stick**. Cook in **50 g (2 oz) butter** for 10 minutes.

2 Drain and add a **425 g (14 oz) can artichoke hearts**, cover and cook for about 3 minutes. Stir in **1 litre (1¾ pints) vegetable stock, 1 tablespoon lemon juice** and **1 tablespoon chopped dill** and cook, covered, for 15 minutes. Purée the soup in batches, transfer to a saucepan and reheat gently.

3 Mix **15 g (½ oz) plain flour** with **150 ml (¼ pint) vegetable stock**. Stir into the soup. Add **2 tablespoons chopped dill**, season with **salt and pepper**, then stir in **150 ml (¼ pint) single cream**. **serves 4**

NUTRITIONAL CONTENT PER 100 G COOKED: energy 8 kcals I **protein** 1 g I **carbohydrates** 1 g I **fat** 0 g I **fibre** 0 g I **folate** 21 mcg I **potassium** 140 mg I **calcium** 19 mg

149

NUTRITIONAL CONTENT PER 100 G RAW: energy 42 kcals | protein 4 g | carbohydrates 4 g | fat 1 g | fibre 4 g | vitamin C 215 mg | folate 135 mcg | vitamin E 1 mg | potassium 450 mg

Brussels sprouts

Resembling miniature cabbages, Brussels sprouts are one of the top brassicas (a group including broccoli, kale, cabbage and cauliflower) for their content of **cancer-fighting phytonutrients**. These work by neutralizing and then removing cancer-causing substances from the body and by deactivating the oestrogens responsible for hormone-related cancers. Sprouts are, therefore, particularly good for preventing digestive and colorectal cancers, and ovarian and breast cancers.

Brussels sprouts are a top source of the antioxidants, especially vitamins A and C, that are useful for keeping the body disease free. In addition, the carotenoids lutein and zeaxanthin help to maintain healthy vision.

During early pregnancy sprouts are useful for their **folic acid**, a vitamin that also helps protect the heart.

The good quantity of fibre in sprouts means they are great for the digestive system and help prevent diseases such as diverticulosis. The fibre can also help **reduce blood cholesterol** levels.

✱ **storing and serving** Keep sprouts in the refrigerator for 1–2 days or they will quickly turn yellow. Boil, braise, microwave or steam sprouts. Cut a cross into the end of large ones to speed up the cooking process, which should be short to prevent nutrient loss.

Brussels sprouts with chestnuts

1 Trim **750 g (1½ lb) Brussels sprouts** and cook in lightly salted boiling water for 10–12 minutes or until tender.

2 Meanwhile, drain a **200 g (7 oz) can chestnuts** into a saucepan, add enough **vegetable stock** to cover and heat gently.

3 Drain the sprouts and the chestnuts. Stir the chestnuts into the sprouts with **15 g (½ oz) butter** and season with **salt and pepper. serves 4–5**

151

chicory and endive

Chicory and endive belong to two closely-related botanical families but are different plants. The chicory family includes the red chicories and Belgian endive and the endive family has broad- and curly-leaved varieties, including frisée and the Batavian endive, which is also known as escarole.

Chicory and endive encourage the growth of 'good' bacteria in the gut, helping to prevent indigestion and disease, and they **improve the body's absorption of nutrients**. They stimulate the appetite, which is good for anyone recovering from illness.

Terpenoids, plant enzymes, help to improve the body's detoxification ability. They also help maintain kidney health and increase urine output.

Both greens are a good source of vitamins A (beta-carotene) and C. They also contain **calcium**, good for helping prevent osteoporosis, and **folic acid**, excellent during pregnancy.

✱ storing and serving Keep chicory and endive in the refrigerator. Usually served as leafy salad greens, they may be briefly baked, steamed or sautéed and served as a main or side dish.

endive and avocado salad

1 Tear ½ **head of curly endive** into pieces and put them in a salad bowl with a **bunch of watercress** separated into sprigs.

2 Halve **2 avocados**, remove the stones and slice the flesh into a bowl. Pour **6 tablespoons French dressing** over the avocados and toss gently until the slices are completely coated.

3 Add the dressed avocado to the endive leaves and toss together.
serves 6

NUTRITIONAL CONTENT PER 100 G ENDIVE, RAW: energy 13 kcals | **protein** 2 g | **carbohydrates** 1 g | **fat** 0 g | **fibre** 2 g | **vitamin C** 12 mg | **carotene** 440 mcg | **potassium** 380 mg

153

honey

A powerful **natural antiseptic** often used for coughs and sore throats, honey also has **antibacterial properties** so is good for stomach upsets.

For those suffering from pollen-triggered hay fever, naturopaths recommend a daily dose of unprocessed organic honey, including honeycomb wax, to build a resistance to pollen. Daily consumption of honey also increases the body's levels of antioxidants, which protect against free-radical-inflicted cellular damage.

Honey is a better sweetener than refined sugar for diabetics as it has less effect on blood sugar levels. It may also help **reduce levels of blood cholesterol** and of homocysteine, which is a risk factor for heart disease.

Use honey in moderation as it is high in calories, and never feed it to babies under one year old because their digestive systems will be unable to deal with it.

✱ storing and serving Raw, unprocessed honey direct from the hive is more nutritious than that bought in the supermarket, which has had many of its phyto-nutrients destroyed by heat treatment. Keep honey in a cool, dark cupboard and use it in place of sugar, but halve the quantity required as it is twice as sweet.

honey and yogurt with prune purée

1 Put **250 g (8 oz) ready-to-eat pitted prunes** in a saucepan with the juice and finely grated rind of **1 lemon** and **8 tablespoons cold water**. Cover and simmer for 6–8 minutes, then blend the mix to a coarse purée.

2 Spoon the purée into 4 glasses and add a layer of **2–3 tablespoons clear honey** to each. Divide **450 g (14½ oz) natural yogurt** among the glasses, then sprinkle each with **½ tablespoon crunchy muesli**. Serve immediately. **serves 4**

NUTRITIONAL CONTENT PER 100 G (1 TBSP = 25 G): energy 288 kcals | **protein** 0 g | **carbohydrates** 76 g | **fat** 0 g | **fibre** 0 g | **potassium** 35 mg | **calcium** 8 mg | **magnesium** 2 mg

NUTRITIONAL CONTENT PER 100 G: energy 266 kcals | protein 0 g | carbohydrates 69 g | fat 0 g | fibre 0 g | potassium 1460 mg | calcium 210 mg | magnesium 240 mg | iron 4.7 mg

molasses

A dark, thick, sweet syrup extracted from sugar cane, molasses is packed with all the nutrients missing from refined sugar: B vitamins, **calcium**, **iron**, **potassium**, magnesium and copper. Blackstrap molasses is the most nutritious type. Its bittersweet flavour varies greatly according to brand, so experiment until you find one you like that has not been processed with sulphur.

Molasses is an iron-rich food – one tablespoon contains more than three times the iron found in an egg – so it is great for building red blood cells, increasing energy and preventing fatigue and anaemia. A tablespoon of molasses also contains more calcium than a glass of milk and more potassium than almost any other food. Molasses is therefore great for bone health and preventing osteoporosis.

Molasses keeps skin and hair looking healthy, and a recent study from Harvard-affiliated McLean Hospital suggests a compound called uridine, found in molasses, may be helpful for preventing depression.

✱ storing and serving Store molasses, tightly sealed, at room temperature or in the refrigerator for up to six months. Try adding to soups, baked beans, meat stews, gingerbread or milk.

fig and molasses cake bars

1 Beat together **125 g (4 oz) unsalted butter**, **50 g (2 oz) raw cane caster sugar** and **3 tablespoons molasses**. Slowly add **3 beaten eggs**.

2 Add **50 g (2 oz) roughly chopped hazelnuts**, **1 teaspoon vanilla extract**, **175 g (6 oz) self-raising flour**, **1 teaspoon baking powder** and ½ **teaspoon ground cinnamon** and mix thoroughly.

3 Stir in **125 g (4 oz) dried ready-to-eat figs**, chopped. Spoon the mixture into a greased and lined 18 x 28 cm (7 x 11 inch) cake tin and bake in a preheated oven, 180°C (350°F), Gas Mark 4, for 20 minutes. Cut into bars. **makes 14**

157

NUTRITIONAL CONTENT PER 100 G PITTED IN BRINE: **energy** 103 kcals | **protein** 1 g | **carbohydrates** 0 g | **fat** 11 g | **fibre** 4 g | **potassium** 91 mg | **calcium** 61 mg | **magnesium** 22 mg

olives and olive oil

The low incidence of serious disease among and longevity of Mediterranean populations is attributed to certain key foods, among them olives and olive oil, which is made from crushed and pressed olives.

The health-boosting properties of olives and olive oil are due to the **'good' monounsaturated fatty acids** and many antioxidants. Eating a small handful of olives a day or using olive oil in place of other fats is highly protective towards the heart thanks to the various compounds that help **reduce blood cholesterol** levels and blood pressure and prevent blood clots.

The specific monounsaturated fats in olives and olive oil are thought to help protect against cancer, particularly breast cancer, and phenols are believed to protect against bowel cancer.

The monounsaturates in olive oil may also help relieve inflammatory conditions, including rheumatoid arthritis and asthma, and help maintain the memory areas of the brain.

✱ **storing and serving** Store both olives and olive oil away from heat and light. Olives can be served as a snack or used to flavour pizzas, pasta sauces or salads. Use virgin olive oil for cooking and extra virgin for drizzling and for salad dressings.

sweet oat cakes

1 Mix together **250 g (8 oz) rolled oats**, **50 g (2 oz) sesame seeds**, **3 tablespoons poppy seeds** and a **pinch of salt**. Pour in **100 ml (3½ fl oz) boiling water**, **2 tablespoons clear honey** and **7 tablespoons olive oil** and stir to form a soft dough.

2 Shape the dough into 20 balls the size of a walnut. Place them on nonstick baking sheets and flatten them with the palm of your hand to make 8 cm (3½ inch) rounds. Bake in a preheated oven, 180°C (350°F), Gas Mark 4, for about 15 minutes until golden.

3 Leave to cool on a wire rack and serve with a wedge of cheese and a bunch of grapes. **makes 20**

soya and tofu

Although soya has been a major food plant in the Far East for thousands of years, it has become important in the West in only the last few decades. The main soya-based product is tofu (bean curd), made from the 'milk' of crushed soya beans. Soya milk is useful for those allergic to dairy products, and soy sauce, made from fermented soya beans, is essential in oriental cuisine.

Soya offers protection against cancer, heart disease and osteoporosis. This is due mainly to the protein and fibre content, which **lowers blood cholesterol levels** and keeps the digestive system healthy, and to the phyto-oestrogens called isoflavones. These plant hormones seem to protect against hormone-related cancers. Isoflavones can help relieve the symptoms of the menopause and premenstrual syndrome (PMS).

Soya is an excellent source of protein and, unlike most animal proteins, lowers blood pressure and cholesterol levels. Its **omega-3 fatty acids** improve heart muscle function.

✱ **storing and serving** Fresh soya beans are not widely available. Use dried beans soaked and cooked in soups and casseroles or sprout them to make bean sprouts. Use silken tofu in dressings and dips, and soft or firm tofu in cooking and smoothies.

peach and tofu smoothie

1 Roughly chop **50 g (2 oz) dried ready-to-eat peaches** in a blender with **75 g (3 oz) soft tofu**. Add a little juice from **300 ml (½ pint) chilled apple juice** and blend to a smooth puree.

2 Add the remaining apple juice and blend again until frothy. Pour into a tall glass, add ice cubes and serve. **serves 1–2**

161

milk

Although it contains high-quality protein, cow's milk is best known for its **calcium** content. Working together with the phosphorous and vitamins D and K in milk, calcium promotes the development of strong bones and teeth. An iron-binding protein in milk, lactoferrin, can help prevent and even reverse osteoporosis.

Young children need whole milk for development, but adults are advised to consume milk with a reduced fat content. Such milk actually has more calcium than whole milk.

Cow's milk supports healthy thyroid function thanks to its **iodine** content, and studies have revealed that it helps reduce the risk of gout.

A calcium-rich diet is associated with fat loss so slimmers may benefit from an increased intake of low-fat dairy foods while following a reduced-calorie diet.

People who are allergic to cow's milk often tolerate **goat's milk**. It offers the same main health benefits as cow's milk.

✱ storing and serving Milk should be kept in the refrigerator and used within a few days of opening.

milk junket with rhubarb

1 Gently heat **1 vanilla pod** in **600 ml (1 pint) milk** until warm. Stir in **1 tablespoon raw cane sugar**.

2 Remove the pan from the heat. Scrape out the vanilla pod seeds and add them to the milk. Stir **10 drops rennet** into the milk. and pour the mixture into a large bowl. Allow to cool and transfer to the refrigerator to set.

3 Roughly chop **750 g (1½ lb) rhubarb** and cook with the juice and grated rind of **1 orange**. Add **2 tablespoons raw cane sugar** and cook for 6–8 minutes, until the rhubarb has softened. Leave to cool and serve with a spoonful of junket and **toasted almonds. serves 4–6**

NUTRITIONAL CONTENT PER 100 ML SEMI-SKIMMED: energy 46 kcals I **protein** 3 g I **carbohydrates** 5 g I **fat** 2 g I **fibre** 0 g I **vitamin C** 1 mg I **potassium** 150 mg I **calcium** 120 mg

163

live yogurt

Yogurt is made by adding bacterial cultures to milk. It contains plenty of nutrients, including **calcium**, but is particularly revered for its live bacteria. The bacteria in live yogurt, *Lactobacillus bulgaricus* and *Streptococcus thermophilus*, together with other probiotics, support the friendly bacteria in the intestine. A daily helping of yogurt therefore helps **protect the digestive system** and fight against gastroenteritis, diarrhoea and food poisoning.

Live yogurt is useful for restoring the bacterial balance in the gut after taking conventional anti-biotics. It can also help prevent and treat ulcers caused by the *Helicobater pylori* bacterium. It can also help counter yeast infections and help reduce bad breath and keep the mouth healthy.

The calcium in yogurt is good for healthy bones and teeth. The beneficial bacteria in yogurt is killed by pasteurization so organic yogurt is the best choice.

✱ storing and serving Use yogurt in dips, dressings and sauces, in cooking, cake mixtures, smoothies and as a topping instead of cream.

blueberry and blackberry yogurt syllabub

1 Gently heat **125 g (4 oz) blackberries** for 2–3 minutes until the juice begins to run out. Remove from the heat and stir in **125 g (4 oz) blueberries**.

2 Whisk **150 ml (¼ pint) whipping cream** with **1–2 tablespoons clear honey** until softly peaking, then stir in **1 tablespoon orange liqueur**. Fold in **300 ml (½ pint) natural yogurt**.

3 Spoon the berries and their juice into 4 bowls and top with the yogurt mixture. Sprinkle over **1 tablespoon toasted flaked almonds** and refrigerate for 1–2 hours before serving. **serves 4**

NUTRITIONAL CONTENT PER 100 G PLAIN LOW-FAT: energy 56 kcals | **protein** 5 g | **carbohydrates** 8 g | **fat** 1 g | **fibre** 0 g | **potassium** 250 mg | **calcium** 190 mg | **magnesium** 19 mg

NUTRITIONAL CONTENT PER MEDIUM EGG: energy 70 kcals | protein 6 g |
carbohydrates 0 g | fat 5 g | fibre 0 g | potassium 65 mg | calcium 29 g | magnesium 6 g

eggs

Eating high-cholesterol foods like eggs was once thought to raise cholesterol levels in the body. It is now known that it is the foods that are high in saturated fat – meats, pastry and high-fat cheese, for example – rather than dietary cholesterol that raise blood cholesterol levels and increase the risk of heart attacks. Indeed, eating eggs may offer some protection against heart disease, breast cancer and eye problems.

One study suggests that eating an egg each day may give teenage girls additional protection against breast cancer in later life, thanks to the presence of amino acids, B vitamins, vitamins A, D and E, **iodine, selenium, phosphorus** and two **vision-protecting carotenoids**, lutein and zeaxanthin.

Pregnant and nursing women, young children and the elderly should avoid eating lightly cooked or raw eggs (as in homemade mayonnaise and uncooked desserts like mousses) because of the risk of food poisoning from salmonella. Pasteurized eggs are the safest option for this group, as pasteurizing kills the bacteria.

✱ **storing and serving** Eat eggs before their 'use by' date. Salmonella bacteria multiply with age so the fresher the egg the better. An excellent source of protein, eggs are ideal for any meal.

watercress and mushroom frittata

1 Slice **250 g (8 oz) mushrooms** and sauté in **20 g (¾ oz) butter**, stirring occasionally, for 3 minutes.

2 Meanwhile, combine **6 beaten eggs** with **5 tablespoons grated Parmesan**, a **bunch of watercress** (tough stems removed) and plenty of **pepper**. Add to the mushrooms and mix gently.

3 Reduce the heat and cook until the egg mixture is lightly set and the underside golden. Place the pan under a preheated moderate grill to cook the top of the frittata. **serves 3–4**

walnuts

Walnut trees were first domesticated thousands of years ago in northern Iran and Turkey, but today the largest commercial producer of walnuts is California. Walnuts are great for heart health, being excellent sources of monounsaturated fats, omega-6 fats and, unusually, of the **omega-3 fatty acids** found mostly in oily fish. These unsaturated fats help **lower cholesterol levels**, prevent blood clotting and reduce the risk of sudden death from dangerous, abnormal heart rhythms.

The omega-3 fats in walnuts, which affect levels of the mood-altering brain chemical serotonin, make them useful for dealing with depression. They also contain melatonin, which aids the body's natural sleep patterns so they may help deal with insomnia.

Walnuts are good for boosting energy levels, but be aware that they are highly calorific if you need to watch your weight.

* storing and serving The oils in nuts means they can go stale quite quickly, so always check the 'use by' dates on packaged walnuts and choose fresh walnuts in their shells where possible. Use walnuts raw as a snack, in breakfast cereals, salads, cakes and breads.

walnut and sunflower seed snacks

1 Mix together **4 tablespoons sunflower seeds** and **25 g (1 oz) sesame seeds**, spread over a baking sheet and toast under a preheated grill for 2–3 minutes.

2 Mix with **250 g (8 oz) roughly chopped walnuts** and **1 tablespoon raisins**. While the seeds are still warm, mix in **3 tablespoons set honey**. Divide the mixture into walnut-sized portions and, with damp hands, firmly press into balls.

3 Place the balls on baking parchment. Leave to cool and dry for 3–4 hours or overnight. **makes 24**

NUTRITIONAL CONTENT PER 100 G NO SHELLS: energy 688 kcals | **protein** 15 g | **carbohydrates** 3 g | **fat** 69 g | **fibre** 6 g | **vitamin E** 3.83 mg | **potassium** 450 mg | **magnesium** 160 mg

Brazil nuts

Brazil nuts are very high in fat (although most of this is the 'good', unsaturated kind) and so should be eaten sparingly. However, they are by far the best food source of the antioxidant **selenium**. A trace mineral, selenium protects the body against free radicals and has an **anti-cancer** function.

Because of their selenium content, Brazil nuts may also be useful in protecting against prostate problems, which commonly affect men from the age of 40 up. In addition, eating Brazil nuts may raise spirits as selenium affects mood, and low selenium levels can lead to irritability, depression and fatigue.

These nuts are a good source of protein for vegetarians and vegans because, weight for weight, they contain as much protein as eggs.

✱ **storing and serving** Keep unshelled nuts in a cool place for no more than a couple of months. Shelled nuts should be transferred to a sealed container in the refrigerator to prevent them from going stale. Use raw as a snack or mixed with breakfast cereal or cook them in a range of sweet or savoury dishes.

Chickpea cakes

1 Chop **250 g (8 oz) Brazil nuts**. Drain 2 **425 g (14 oz) cans organic chickpeas**. Blend nuts and chickpeas until smooth. Chop **1 small onion** and mix with **25 g (1 oz) sunflower seeds** and **1 tablespoon chopped parsley**.

2 Beat **1 egg** with **salt and pepper**, combine with chickpea mixture and blend together. Using a large tablespoon press the mixture into 8 or 16 flat patties.

3 Dip each patty in **lightly beaten egg** and coat with **125 g (4 oz) wholemeal breadcrumbs**. Chill for 4 hours or overnight, then shallow-fry in **vegetable oil** until golden-brown. Serve with vegetables and a tomato sauce. **serves 4**

NUTRITIONAL CONTENT PER 100 G WHOLE: energy 682 kcals | protein 14 g | carbohydrates 3 g | fat 68 g | fibre 8 g | vitamin E 7.18 mg | selinium 1530 mcg | potassium 660 mg

171

hazelnuts

Hazelnuts, also known as filberts and cobnuts, are one of the richest dietary sources of **vitamin E**. This powerful antioxidant helps neutralize free radicals, which are responsible for cell destruction and disease. It is also essential for healthy muscles and supports the body's red blood cells, preventing anaemia.

Hazelnuts are a good source of manganese, which plays a role in blood sugar regulation and may help reduce symptoms of pre-menstrual stress (PMS), and the anti-oxidant **zinc**, which, eaten regularly, can offer protection against cancer, heart disease and premature ageing.

Other heart-protective nutrients in hazelnuts include omega-6 oils, plant sterols and fibre, all of which help **lower blood cholesterol** levels. Because they are a rich source of fibre, hazelnuts are good for the digestive system. The fibre helps the digestive tract function smoothly, reducing the risk of bowel cancer.

✱ **storing and serving** For maximum nutrients and flavour buy unprocessed hazelnuts. Shell and eat as they are or roast gently to release more flavour. Eat as a snack, add to salads or use in cakes and biscuits.

grapefruit and prawn salad

1 Halve **2 large pink grapefruit** and loosen the segments but leave them in the skins.

2 Sprinkle a **pinch of chilli flakes, 1 teaspoon honey** and a **pinch of paprika** over the segments and grill for 5–6 minutes. Spoon out the grapefruit segments and add to a bowl with **250 g (8 oz) cooked peeled prawns, 75 g (3 oz) beansprouts** and **1 tablespoon chopped fresh coriander**. Dry-fry **75 g (3 oz) hazelnuts**, chop and mix in the bowl.

3 Mix **2 tablespoons lemon juice, 1 tablespoon olive oil, 1 teaspoon honey, salt and pepper**, pour over the salad and toss. **serves 4**

NUTRITIONAL CONTENT PER 100 G SHELLED NUTS: energy 650 kcals | protein 14 g | carbohydrates 6 g | fat 64 g | fibre 9 g | vitamin E 25 mg | zinc 2.2 mg | manganese 4.9 mg

173

NUTRITIONAL CONTENT PER 100 G ROASTED, SALTED CASHEWS: energy 611 kcals
| **protein** 21 g | **carbohydrates** 19 g | **fat** 51 g | **fibre** 3 g | **iron** 6.2 mg | **copperl** 2.04 mg

cashews

If you are prone to anaemia and fatigue, eating cashews regularly – for both their **copper and iron** content – will help build the red blood cells your body needs. They contain roughly twice as much iron as almonds, walnuts and hazelnuts. Eat them with a vitamin C-rich fruit or fruit juice to increase your body's absorption of the iron.

The high levels of magnesium in cashews are important for strengthening bones, hair and teeth. They are a good source of the mineral **zinc**, which is essential for healthy skin, hair and nails, healing wounds and improving immunity. In addition, they contain beta-carotene, which the body converts to vitamin A, an antioxidant vitamin essential for immune health and building resistance to disease.

Like all nuts, cashews are a good source of protein for vegetarians.

✱ **storing and serving** Cashews are always sold shelled because the shells contain an oily liquid that can cause the skin to blister. Keep them in the refrigerator for up to six months. If you eat cashews as a snack avoid too many salted ones, especially if you have high blood pressure. Add raw cashews to breakfast cereal or use them in salads or stir-fries.

cashew chicken

1 Heat **250 ml (8 fl oz) chicken stock** in a saucepan. Cube and add **400 g (13 oz) chicken breast** and bring to the boil. Simmer for 5 minutes. Remove chicken and set aside.

2 Add. **2 tablespoons yellow bean sauce.** Cook for a couple of minutes. Slice and add **200 g (7 oz) carrots** and **200 g (7 oz) bamboo shoots**. Cook for another couple of minutes.

3 Return the chicken to the pan, bring the sauce to the boil and thicken with **1 teaspoon cornflour** mixed with **2 tablespoons water**.

4 Stir in **200 g (7 oz) cashew nuts** and **1 shredded spring onion** before serving with boiled white rice. **serves 2**

almonds

One of the earliest nut trees to be cultivated, almonds were being grown in the Mediterranean by 3000 BC.

These nuts are rich in the monounsaturated fats that help protect against heart disease by **lowering blood cholesterol levels**. Almond skins contain flavonoids, which work in tandem with almonds' antioxidant **vitamin E** and can help prevent clogged arteries.

Vitamin E is also protective against cancer, as are two phytochemicals found in almonds, quercetin and kaempferol, which can suppress tumour growth.

Weight for weight, almonds are richer in protein than eggs so are a good choice for vegetarians, although their protein needs 'completing' with legumes.

Almonds are also particularly high in **calcium** – 50 g (2 oz) almonds contain more calcium than half a cup of milk – which the body needs for strengthening bones and teeth. Almonds can, therefore, be a good for people who are intolerant of dairy products.

✱ storing and serving Almonds are most nutritious when eaten raw and unsalted. The oils in nuts give them a limited shelf-life and almonds can go rancid very easily. If possible, buy them in their shells.

almond macaroons

1 Mix together **125 g (4 oz) ground almonds** and **150 g (5 oz) caster sugar**. Whisk together **½ teaspoon almond extract** and **2 large egg whites** until stiff. Fold in the ground almond mixture.

2 Place teaspoonfuls of the mixture on lined baking sheets, leaving spaces between them so they can expand slightly. Cook in a preheated oven, 180°C (350°F), Gas Mark 4, for 15 minutes, until slightly firm.

3 Remove the macaroons from the oven and leave to cool for 5 minutes. Lift them off the baking parchment with a palette knife and leave to cool completely. **makes about 16**

NUTRITIONAL CONTENT PER 100 G NO SHELLS: energy 612 kcals I **protein** 21 g I **carbohydrates** 7 g I **fat** 56 g I **fibre** 13 g I **vitamin E** 24 mg I **potassium** 870 mg I **calcium** 240 mg

oats

Countless studies have shown that a daily helping of oats is **heart protective** because the soluble fibre in oats sticks to 'bad' cholesterol and removes it from the body, thereby preventing it from clogging arteries.

Oats are a particularly good food at the start of the day because their fibre content means that sugars are released slowly into the bloodstream, providing energy without upsetting blood sugar levels.

In addition, eating oats reduces the risk of cancer because of the presence of a trace mineral in oats called **selenium**, plant hormones called lignans and the insoluble fibre they contain. Selenium is linked with a reduced risk of bowel and prostate cancers, lignans account for a lowered risk of hormone-related cancers, and the insoluble fibre attacks certain bile acids, making them less toxic and potentially carcinogenic. Selenium may also help ward off depression.

✱ **storing and serving** Oats will keep for a couple of months in an airtight container. Enjoy them raw in muesli or cooked in porridge. They make an ideal coating for fried fish or a crumble topping, or use them for baking muesli bars, flapjacks or biscuits.

blueberry porridge and nuts

1 Gently heat **125 g (4 oz) blueberries** and **1–3 tablespoons unrefined caster sugar** (to taste) for 6 minutes or until the berry juice begins to run. Remove from heat.

2 Put **150 g (5 oz) rolled oats** and **1 litre (1¾ pints) milk** in a pan. Add **sugar** to taste and bring to the boil, stirring constantly. Simmer for 6–8 minutes, stirring from time to time, and add extra milk if liked.

3 Serve the porridge topped with blueberries, **3 tablespoons toasted nuts**, a little **soft dark brown sugar** and **1–2 tablespoons toasted wheatgerm**. Pour some **buttermilk (or yogurt)** over the porridge and serve. **serves 4**

NUTRITIONAL CONTENT PER 100 G ROLLED, RAW: energy 400 kcals | **protein** 12 g | **carbohydrates** 73 g | **fat** 9 g | **fibre** 6 g | **potassium** 370 mg | **magnesium** 110 mg | **selenium** 3 mcg

sunflower seeds

Because they contain the goodness necessary to germinate a new plant, all seeds are a concentrated source of nutrients. Sunflower seeds (they are technically fruits, known as achenes) are particularly health-boosting for their rich **vitamin E** content, and their **selenium** and magnesium.

The antioxidant vitamin E and the trace mineral, selenium, work especially well together to **protect against cancer**. Sunflower seeds may benefit those suffering from rheumatoid arthritis and asthma as they have **anti-inflammatory** properties.

Sunflower seeds are high in the beneficial and essential unsaturated fats (omega-6). They also contain cholesterol-lowering compounds called phytosterols, vitamin E, which helps disarm free radicals and magnesium, which helps reduce high blood pressure.

✻ storing and serving The fat in sunflower seeds can turn them rancid so keep them in an airtight container, preferably in the refrigerator. Dry-frying or roasting sunflower seeds enhances their flavour. Snack on them, add them to stir-fries and salads, or use them in home baking.

savoury seed snacks

1 Put **250 g (8 oz) assorted seeds** (including sunflower, pumpkin, hemp, flaxseed (linseed) and sesame seeds) into a bowl, add **2 tablespoons tamari sauce** and stir until all the seeds are covered with the sauce.

2 Drain the seeds through a fine sieve, then dry-fry in a hot pan for a few minutes until golden-brown. Remove the pan from the heat, lift out the seeds on to a piece of kitchen paper and allow to cool. **serves 4**

NUTRITIONAL CONTENT PER 100 G RAW: energy 582 kcals I **protein** 20 g I **carbohydrates** 19 g I **fat** 48 g I **fibre** 6 g I **vitamin E** 38 mg I **magnesium** 270 mg I **selenium** 49 mcg

pumpkin seeds

Men of middle age and beyond would do well to snack regularly on pumpkin seeds as they are an excellent food for maintaining prostate health and reducing the risk of prostate cancer. This is believed to be due to the high levels of **zinc** and to certain compounds in pumpkin seed oil. Zinc also supports bone mineral density, which is as important for older men as it is for post-menopausal women.

Pumpkin seeds make an energizing snack because of their energy-producing zinc and their iron, which boosts blood cells. They also contribute to a healthy heart thanks to their essential **omega-3 fatty acids** and **cholesterol-lowering compounds** called phytosterols.

Eating pumpkin seeds may help to lift the spirits because of their zinc, B vitamins and omega-3 fats, all of which can help prevent depression.

✱ storing and serving Pumpkin seeds are available roasted or raw. Keep them in the refrigerator because of their oil content. Eat as a snack, add to cereals, soups, casseroles and salads, or use them in home baking. Pumpkin seed oil can be used to dress salads or added to protein drinks.

pumpkin seed dip

1 Dry-fry **175 g (6 oz) pumpkin seeds** over a moderate heat for 5–10 minutes. Shake the pan and turn them as they pop and go golden-brown. Remove the pan from the heat and allow to cool.

2 Grind the seeds coarsely in a food processor and skin, deseed and dice **3 large tomatoes**. Add **2 finely chopped garlic cloves**, **3–5 chopped spring onions**, **½ teaspoon ground cumin**, the juice of **½ lime** and **3 tablespoons tomato purée** and blend until the mixture is smooth. **serves 4**

NUTRITIONAL CONTENT PER 100 G RAW: energy 569 kcals I **protein** 24 g I **carbohydrates** 15 g I **fat** 46 g I **fibre** 5 g I **potassium** 820 mg I **magnesium** 270 mg I **zinc** 6.6 mg

sesame seeds

Widely used in Middle Eastern cooking, sesame seeds are the main ingredient in tahini, a paste used to make hummus. Of all the nuts and seeds, sesame seeds have the highest content of phytosterols, plant compounds that are believed to **reduce blood cholesterol** levels, **boost the immune system** and reduce the risk of certain types of cancer.

Sesame seeds are a good source of **calcium**, so a useful alternative for anyone allergic to dairy products. They may also provide some relief from rheumatoid arthritis because of their high levels of copper, which has **anti-inflammatory** properties. The magnesium in sesame seeds relaxes blood vessels and may benefit migraine sufferers.

Cooking with sesame seed oil can lower blood pressure thanks to an antioxidant called sesamin.

✱ storing and serving Once hulled, sesame seeds should be kept in the refrigerator to prevent the oils turning rancid. Sprinkle over vegetables or salads or use in home baking.

honeyed granola

1 Warm **3 tablespoons sunflower oil** and **3 tablespoons thick honey** in a saucepan.

2 Stir in **2 tablespoons golden flaxseeds, 2 tablespoons sesame seeds, 50 g (2 oz) roughly chopped hazelnuts, 50 g (2 oz) barley flakes, 50 g (2 oz) rye flakes, 50 g (2 oz) millet flakes**.

3 Spread the mixture evenly over a lightly oiled baking sheet with edges. Bake in a preheated oven, 180°C (350°F), Gas Mark 4, for 8–10 minutes, stirring the mixture halfway through cooking.

3 Leave to cool then transfer to a storage jar. Store in a cool place for up to 2 weeks. **serves 6**

NUTRITIONAL CONTENT PER 100 g: energy 598 kcals | **protein** 18 g | **carbohydrates** 1 g | **fat** 58 g | **fibre** 8 g | **calcium** 670 mg | **potassium** 570 mg | **magnesium** 370 mg | **copper** 1.46 mg

185

flaxseed

Also known as linseed, these are the seeds of the flax plant. The largest plant source of essential **omega-3 fatty acids**, flaxseed is hugely important for vegetarians because the other main dietary source is oily fish. These fats thin the blood and, together with fibre, help **lower blood cholesterol** levels, which explains the role of flaxseed and flaxseed oil in protecting against heart disease.

Flaxseed also **helps combat cancer**, especially breast and bowel cancers. This is due partly to lignans, anti-oestrogen plant compounds that are highly protective against hormone-related cancers, and partly to fibre. This fibre is great for the digestive system, speeding potentially carcinogenic substances out of the body, and it also makes flaxseed a good remedy for constipation and of help to sufferers of irritable bowel syndrome (IBS).

✱ **storing and serving** Flaxseed is available whole or ground, but the nutrients are more easily absorbed when ground. Store whole flaxseed in an airtight container; keep ground flaxseed and flaxseed oil refrigerated. Add ground flaxseed to juices, smoothies, yogurt, cereal, breads and biscuits. Don't heat flaxseed oil – use it in salad dressings or drinks. Industrial blends of linseed oil are not for internal consumption.

flaxseed crackers

1 Sift together **100 g (3½ oz) wholemeal flour**, 100 g (3½ oz) **plain white flour**, ½ teaspoon **baking powder** and ½ **teaspoon bicarbonate of soda**, adding any bran left in the sieve. Stir in **3 tablespoons golden flaxseeds** and a **pinch of salt**. Rub in **50 g (2 oz) butter** and **3 tablespoons olive oil** and add about **1 tablespoon water** to make a smooth dough.

2 Roll out the dough to about 5 mm (¼ inch) thick. Cut out rounds and transfer to a greased baking sheet. Bake in a preheated oven, 200°C (400°F), Gas Mark 6, for 15 minutes. Cool on a wire rack. **makes about 20**

sardines and mackerel

Oily fish, such as sardines and mackerel, are particularly beneficial due to their **omega-3 fatty acids**, which are vital for brain function and a healthy heart. According to the American Heart Association, eating two portions of oily fish weekly can prevent heart attacks.

Omega-3 fatty acids are also linked with reducing the severity of inflammatory disorders and may be useful for sufferers of asthma, rheumatoid arthritis and psoriasis.

Sardines and mackerel provide vitamin D, which is important for strong bones and teeth, and **selenium**, an antioxidant mineral linked with a reduced cancer risk.

Unlike canned tuna, canned sardines and mackerel retain their beneficial oils and match the fresh fish for nutritional content. Fish canned with their bones (which soften during the canning process) are rich in **calcium**, **phosphorus** and fluoride, so are great for maintaining bone health and preventing osteoporosis.

✱ **storing and serving** Keep fresh fish in the refrigerator or, if it has not been frozen previously, in the freezer. Serve mackerel simply with a squeeze of lemon or team it with sharp flavours, such as gooseberry. Sardines are a good fish for the barbecue.

spiced mackerel and celeriac mash

1 Mix **1 teaspoon cumin seeds**, **1 teaspoon crushed black peppercorns** and a **pinch of chilli flakes** and sprinkle over **4 mackerel**, gutted and descaled. Cover. Refrigerate for 2–3 hours.

2 Put the mackerel into an ovenproof dish, stuff the cavities with **dill sprigs** and pour **150 ml (¼ pint) dry cider** over the fish. Loosely cover with foil and bake in a preheated oven, 200°C (400°F), Gas Mark 6, for 15–20 minutes.

3 Peel and dice **375 g (12 oz) celeriac** and boil for 5 minutes. Peel and dice **750 g (1½ lb) potatoes**, then add for 15 minutes. Drain and mash with **milk** and **olive oil**. **serves 4**

NUTRITIONAL CONTENT PER 100 G SARDINES (MACKEREL): energy 165 (223) kcals I protein 21 (19) g I carbohydrates 0 (0) g I fat 9 (16) g I fibre 0 (0) g I selenium 34 (30) mcg

tuna

Although tuna is a great source of high-quality protein and vitamins, its essential **omega-3 fatty acids** are the main health-boosters. However, this applies to fresh tuna only. Canned tuna has much of its omega-3 content removed in the canning process.

Unlike artery-clogging saturated animal fats, unsaturated fish oils are great for heart health. They improve the ratio between 'good' and 'bad' cholesterol, make the blood less likely to clot, reduce blood pressure and help prevent irregular heart rhythms. Tuna is also a good source of folic acid and vitamin B_6, which together neutralize excessive levels of homocysteine, the heart attack-causing amino acid.

Fish oils have **anti-inflammatory** properties. These, combined with tuna's anti-inflammatory biotin and vitamin B_3 (**niacin**) help rheumatoid arthritis.

Pregnant women should restrict their tuna intake because of foetus-harming mercury levels in the fish.

✱ **storing and serving** Bake, griddle or grill fresh tuna. When you are buying canned tuna, choose fish canned in water rather than in oil or brine.

griddled tuna and tomato sauce

1 Place **4 x 100 g (3½ oz) tuna steaks**, 2 at a time, on a preheated hot griddle, and cook for 3 minutes on each side. Remove and keep warm.

2 Make the tomato sauce by blending together **4 plum tomatoes, 1 teaspoon garlic purée, 1 tablespoon tomato purée** and **1 tablespoon chopped parsley** for 1 minute. Transfer to a saucepan and cook, uncovered, for 10 minutes.

3 Season with **salt and pepper**, spoon over the cooked tuna and serve. **serves 4**

NUTRITIONAL CONTENT PER 100 G: energy 136 kcals | protein 24 g | carbohydrates 0 g | fat 5 g | fibre 0 g | vitamin B_6 0.38 mg | potassium 400 mg | magnesium 33 mg | selenium 57 mcg

191

192

NUTRITIONAL CONTENT PER 100 G RAW FILLET: energy 182 kcals | protein 18 g | carbohydrates 0 g | fat 12 g | fibre 0 g | potassium 310 mg | calcium 27 mg | selenium 20 mcg

salmon

All fish contain the beneficial **omega-3 fatty acids** that are essential for the body's function, but oily fish contain far more than white fish, and salmon contains more than most.

Research has shown that fish oils are highly beneficial for the heart and help to fight cancer, particularly breast and bowel cancers. (Salmon's anti-cancer mineral **selenium** may enhance this protective action.)

Moreover, fish oils are 'brain food', and including salmon in the diet may improve memory and brain function and help prevent the mental deterioration seen in diseases such as Alzheimer's. It may also help with depression as fish oils affect levels of serotonin.

The fish oils can reduce inflammation, so sufferers from asthma, rheumatoid arthritis, lupus and skin conditions, including eczema, may find it helpful to include salmon and other oily fish regularly in their diet.

Canning softens the bones, making them edible, and these provide **calcium**, **fluoride** and **phosphorus**, good for helping prevent osteoporosis.

✳ buying If possible, choose wild and organic salmon over farmed varieties. Leaner and firmer, these fish contain none of the dyes, antibiotics or growth-hormone residues found in many farmed fish.

salmon with herb sauce

1 Cook **4 x 50 g (2 oz) salmon steaks** under a preheated moderate grill for 4 minutes on each side.

2 Make the herb sauce by combining **1 tablespoon chopped basil** and **1 tablespoon chopped tarragon** with **175 g (6 oz) natural yogurt**. Season with **salt and pepper**.

3 Serve the salmon with the sauce and **lemon wedges**. **serves 4**

anchovies

Anchovies, which are small oily fish, are an acquired taste and usually used in only small quantities.

They are a rich source of the beneficial fish oils known as **omega-3 fatty acids**, which **lower blood cholesterol** and blood pressure, thereby reducing the risk of heart disease and strokes.

Anchovies may also be helpful for anyone suffering from depression, because the same omega-3 fats affect levels of the mood-altering 'feel-good' brain chemical serotonin.

Protein-rich, anchovies contain **calcium**, **iron** and **phosphorus** and are a good source of **selenium**, an antioxidant mineral that helps neutralize damaging free radicals, providing some protection against cancer.

Avoid anchovies if you suffer from gout or inflamed joints because the purines they contain increase the level of uric acid in the joints and exacerbate the pain.

✱ storing and serving Most commonly consumed as canned fillets, anchovies are sometimes available fresh or frozen. They are very salty. Rinsing them removes some of the salt (and the oil in which they are canned), but if they are still too salty for your taste, soak them in a little milk for 5 minutes then rinse and pat them dry with kitchen paper.

boiled eggs with anchovy soldiers

1 Boil **4 large eggs** for 4–5 minutes until softly set.

2 Meanwhile, drain the oil and rinse **8 anchovy fillets** and pat dry with kitchen paper. Chop finely then beat into **25 g (1 oz) softened unsalted butter** and season with **pepper**.

3 Spread 4 thick **slices of toast** with the anchovy butter. Cut the toast into fingers and serve with the boiled eggs. **serves 4**

prawns

Prawns, known as shrimp in the USA, are a low-fat, low-calorie protein, and thus perfect food for slimmers. They are high in cholesterol, but it is now known that this has no adverse effect on blood cholesterol levels. On the contrary, the **omega-3 fatty acids** in prawns can help **lower blood cholesterol** levels as well as reducing blood pressure. They make the blood less likely to clot (a risk factor for strokes and heart attack), making prawns a really good food for preventing heart disease. Another cardio-protective nutrient in prawns is **vitamin B$_{12}$**, which regulates the body's levels of the heart attack-causing amino acid, homocysteine.

Eating prawns is good for brain development and function and for dealing with depression, and they may help reduce aggressive tendencies in some people.

Prawns can help reduce the risk of cancer thanks to their levels of the **anti-cancer** mineral **selenium**.

✱ **storing and serving** Prawns vary greatly in size and price, but they all taste much the same. Take care not to refreeze so-called fresh prawns, which have often been frozen at sea for optimum freshness and thawed for sale. Use prawns hot or cold.

Kerala prawn curry

1 Sprinkle ½ **teaspoon ground turmeric** over **500 g (1 lb) large cooked peeled prawns** and set aside.

2 Cut **1 red onion** into fine wedges and deseed and slice **2 green chillies**. Stir-fry in **1 teaspoon vegetable oil** until softened.

3 Add the prawns, **10 curry leaves** (optional) and **100 ml (3½ fl oz) coconut milk** and simmer for 5 minutes. Sprinkle over **2 tablespoons lime juice** and season with **salt and pepper**. Scatter with a few **fresh coriander leaves** and stir once. Serve immediately. **serves 4**

NUTRITIONAL CONTENT PER 100 G BOILED: energy 99 kcals | protein 23 g | carbohydrates 0 g | fat 1 g | fibre 0 g | potassium 260 mg | calcium 110 mg | selenium 45 mcg

197

oysters

Oysters have long been considered an aphrodisiac, probably because they are the richest food source of **zinc**. Zinc is essential for sexual health, particularly men's, because it is required for testosterone and sperm production and may help with infertility or impotence. Thanks to both zinc and **selenium**, oysters are great for prostate health and reducing the risk of prostate cancer.

Oysters contain more selenium than other shellfish. This trace mineral helps protect against bowel cancer.

Oysters are good 'brain food', and their essential **omega-3 fatty acids** are good for heart health. Although rich in cholesterol, oysters are very low in saturated fat, which is the real culprit when it comes to raised blood cholesterol levels and an increased risk of heart attack.

Oysters may be helpful in fighting fatigue and anaemia because of their **blood-boosting iron** content.

✱ **storing and serving** Keep oysters alive until you are ready to cook them by covering them with a damp tea towel in the refrigerator. Use them within a week, discarding any with open shells because these have died. Serve oysters raw or barely cooked, or you can bake, steam, poach, sauté or grill them.

oriental steamed oysters

1 Remove the top shell from **12 shucked oysters**. Strain the juices through a sieve into a small pan. Wipe out any grit from the shells.

2 Slice **2 spring onions** (white parts only), peel and grate **1½ cm (¾ inch) fresh root ginger**, slice **1 small garlic clove** and deseed and slice **1 small red chilli**. Add to **50 ml (2 fl oz) sake**, **2 tablespoons rice vinegar** and **2 teaspoons dark soy sauce** with the oyster juices. Warm gently.

3 Arrange the oysters in a large bamboo steamer, cover and steam for 2 minutes. Put on plates and spoon over the sauce. Serve with **fresh coriander leaves. serves 4**

NUTRITIONAL CONTENT PER 100 G RAW: energy 65 kcals | **protein** 11 g | **carbohydrates** 3 g | **fat** 1 g | **fibre** 0 g | **potassium** 260 mg | **zinc** 59.2 mg | **copper** 7.5 mg | **selenium** 23 mcg | **iron** 5.7 mg

mussels

Like most seafood, mussels are rich in the cardio-protective **omega-3 fatty acids**, which are vital for the body. In addition to protecting the heart and enhancing brain function, omega-3 fats are **anti-inflammatory** agents and may help sufferers from asthma, rheumatoid arthritis, psoriasis and inflammatory bowel disease (IBS).

Including mussels in the diet is especially beneficial for menstruating women and new mothers and for middle-aged and elderly men. This is because mussels are rich in both **iron**, which is good for combating fatigue and anaemia, and **zinc**, which is required for male sexual function and prostate health.

Like a lot of seafood, mussels also contain **iodine**, which is needed for healthy thyroid function, and **vitamin E** and **selenium**, which protect cells and tissues from damage by free radicals and are therefore important for fighting cancer.

✱ **storing and serving** Keep live mussels in the refrigerator covered with a damp tea towel. Use them within a week, discarding any with open shells. Do not overcook mussels as this toughens them. Serve them, in or out of their shells, in seafood soups, stews and salads or simply bake them in their shells.

mussel gratin

1 Heat **4 tablespoons white wine** in a saucepan until bubbling. Clean, debeard and add **500 g (1 lb) mussels**. Cover and cook for 4–5 minutes Drain, reserving cooking juices. Discard any closed shells.

2 Remove the mussels from their shells. Break the shells apart and arrange half of them on a foil-lined grill rack. Place a mussel in each.

3 Blend **75 g (3 oz) crème fraîche** with 4 tablespoons of the cooking juices. Spoon into the shells.

4 Melt **50 g (2 oz) butter** in a frying pan. Stir in **2 crushed garlic cloves, 75 g (3 oz) breadcrumbs, 4 tablespoons chopped mixed herbs** and season. Spoon over the mussels and grill until lightly toasted.
serves 4

scallops

Scallops have heart-protective properties due to their high levels of **omega-3 fatty acids** and vitamin B_{12} and of magnesium and **potassium**, which help regulate blood-pressure levels. Vitamin B_{12} reduces a harmful build-up of the amino acid homocysteine, high levels of which increase the risk of stroke and heart attack.

The omega-3 fatty acids in seafood are unsaturated fats that improve the ratio of 'good' and 'bad' cholesterol. They reduce high blood pressure, make the blood less likely to clot and help regulate the heart beat.

Eating scallops may **improve memory** and protect against age-related dementia. In addition, the protein in scallops and oysters contains the amino acid tyrosine, which produces mentally energizing chemicals that enhance attentiveness and the speed of reactions.

Scallops are also good for protecting against cancer because of their high levels of **anti-cancer selenium**.

✱ storing and serving Scallops are usually sold removed from their shells. They are highly perishable and should be refrigerated and eaten on the day of purchase. Scallops need only a few minutes' cooking or they will become tough.

seared scallops with lime-dressed salad

1 Clean **16 large scallops** and dry them well with kitchen paper to remove excess water. Cook on a preheated hot griddle for 3 minutes on each side.

2 Mix together the grated rind and juice of **2 limes**, **3 tablespoons olive oil** and a **bunch of chopped dill**. Season with **salt and pepper**.

3 Toss a large bag of **mixed salad leaves** in the lime dressing and arrange on 4 plates. Plate the scallops on top and garnish with a little of the dressing. **serves 4**

NUTRITIONAL CONTENT PER 100 G STEAMED NO SHELL: energy 118 kcals I **protein** 23 g I **carbohydrates** 3 g I **fat** 1 g I **fibre** 0 g I **potassium** 240 mg I **magnesium** 38 mg I **zinc** 2.4 mg

203

brown rice

Unlike white rice, which is stripped of its layers and therefore nutrients during processing, brown rice is a natural whole grain with a high fibre content.

Fibre helps the digestive system function efficiently, protecting against bowel cancer by quickly conveying waste matter out of the body. Brown rice also contains the antioxidant **anti-cancer** trace mineral **selenium**, which is protective against bowel and prostate cancers.

Eating brown rice is good for the heart because both the fibre and a compound in its bran (the outer layer) called **orysanol** help reduce the body's levels of 'bad' cholesterol. This cholesterol can clog arteries, resulting in strokes and heart attacks.

The fibre makes brown rice a great source of slow-burning energy and helps stabilize blood sugar levels, so is particularly good for diabetics and athletes.

✱ storing and serving Because its natural oils can turn rancid brown rice is best kept in an airtight container in the refrigerator. Soaking brown rice before use reduces the cooking time. To retain the nutrients, use the same water for cooking, and don't cook with excess water that then has to be drained.

brown rice pudding with sultanas and almonds

1 Rinse **75 g (3 oz) brown rice** and cook for 15 minutes. Drain then bring slowly to the boil with **900 ml (1½ pints) milk** and **25 g (1 oz) soft light brown sugar**.

2 Pour into a buttered, ovenproof 1.2 litre (2 pint) dish. Add **75 g (3 oz) sultanas** and stir. Sprinkle over ½ **teaspoon grated nutmeg** and dot with **15 g (½ oz) butter**.

3 Cook in the centre of a preheated oven, 180°C (350°F), Gas Mark 4, for 1½–2 hours, stirring twice. Sprinkle with chopped **stem ginger** and **flaked almonds**. Serve with crème fraîche. **serves 4–6**

NUTRITIONAL CONTENT PER 100 G BOILED: energy 140 kcals | **protein** 3 g | carbohydrates 32 g | fat 1 g | **fibre** 1.5 g | **potassium** 99 mg | **magnesium** 43 mg | **calcium** 4 mg

205

buckwheat

Often categorized as a grain, buckwheat is actually a seed. Free of gluten, it is suitable for people who suffer with coeliac disease.

The flavonoids in buckwheat help protect against heart disease. These antioxidant compounds, rutin in particular, help prevent blood clots and **reduce levels of blood cholesterol**, as well as lowering high blood pressure. Rutin strengthens and tones blood vessels so can help people suffering from varicose veins.

Buckwheat may help prevent cancer, as it contains rutin and quercetin, together with the free radical-fighting **vitamin E**. Its high fibre content stimulates the digestive tract into removing quickly potentially toxic substances before they can cause harmful tumours.

Buckwheat can help prevent and manage diabetes, because it is a good source of slow-release energy, which stops fluctuating blood sugar levels.

✱ storing and serving Store buckwheat in an airtight container in a cupboard or in the refrigerator. Use ground buckwheat to make a porridge-like breakfast cereal, and serve the whole kernels like rice.

Breton crêpes

1 Lightly beat **2 eggs, 1 tablespoon vegetable oil** and **100 ml (3½ fl oz) beer (or cider).**

2 Sift **125 g (4 oz) buckwheat flour** into a bowl, then gradually add the liquid, whisking to form a smooth batter. Thin with **175 ml (6 fl oz) water** and whisk again. Leave to stand for 10 minutes.

3 Brush a 14 cm (5½ inch) frying pan with **vegetable oil** and heat. Coat the base of the pan with batter and tip from side to side to cover the base before the mixture sets. Cook on each side for 30 seconds, flipping inbetween. Remove the crêpes from the pan, cover and keep warm while you cook the remainder. Serve with ratatouille, if liked. **makes about 15**

NUTRITIONAL CONTENT PER 100 G RAW: energy 364 kcals | **protein** 8 g | **carbohydrates** 85 g | **fat** 2 g | **fibre** 2 g | **potassium** 220 mg | **magnesium** 48 mg | **calcium** 12 mg | **iron** 2 mg

NUTRITIONAL CONTENT PER 100 G RAW: energy 309 kcals | **protein** 14 g |

carbohydrates 56 g | **fat** 5 g | **fibre** 6 g | **vitamin E** 4.87 mg | **magnesium** 210 mg | **manganese** 2.25 mg

quinoa

The ancient Incas regarded quinoa as a sacred food, and each season the emperor was responsible for planting the first seed.

Quinoa is a seed rather than a grain, but it has many of the qualities of grain, being a low-fat, energizing, cancer-preventing, heart-protecting whole food. An excellent source of **complete protein**, on a par with milk, quinoa is great for vegetarians and vegans.

Eating quinoa regularly may assist migraine sufferers because the **magnesium** it contains relaxes blood vessels and improves blood flow. The vitamin B_2 (riboflavin) may help reduce the frequency of attacks.

Whole 'grains' like quinoa have a role in cancer prevention thanks to their high fibre levels, (which help protect against bowel cancer), lignans (plant hormones thought to protect against hormone-related cancers), and free radical-fighting manganese and copper.

Eating quinoa regularly can help keep the heart healthy, as the fibre in this grain lowers cholesterol.

✱ **storing and serving** Store quinoa in an airtight container in a cupboard or in the refrigerator. Rinse well to remove any residue of its inedible coating. Dry-fry quinoa before cooking to enhance its nutty flavour, then cook as you would rice.

quinoa coconut ice cream

1 Put **75 g (3 oz) quinoa seeds** and **175 ml (6 fl oz) rice milk** in a saucepan, bring to the boil and simmer gently for 15 minutes. Beat in **175 ml (6 fl oz) soya milk**. Simmer for another 5 minutes. Add **50 ml (2 fl oz) maple syrup** and **200 ml (7 fl oz) coconut milk** and beat again.

2 Still beating, add **100 ml (3½ fl oz) rapeseed oil**, **1 teaspoon vanilla extract**, **1 tablespoon lemon juice** and **1 chopped banana** and beat until smooth. Transfer to an airtight container and freeze for 12 hours, stirring every hour or two to break up any ice crystals. **serves 4**

wheatgerm

Wheatgerm is the most nutritious part of the wheat grain, yet is discarded in the refining process that makes white flour. A highly concentrated source of nutrients, it contains protein, B vitamins such as **folic acid**, **vitamin E**, **zinc**, **selenium**, **iron** and magnesium.

Because wheatgerm is such a good source of fibre, it can ease constipation and by ensuring the smooth and efficient operation of the digestive tract, it helps prevent bowel cancer. Selenium has effective **anti-cancer** properties, too.

Wheatgerm is a good source of vitamin E, which is linked to a reduced risk of stroke, heart disease and cancer. It is also particularly important for maintaining healthy skin, heart and circulation, nerves, muscles and red blood cells.

The folic acid in wheatgerm helps to protect unborn children from spina bifida. Wheatgerm can also prevent fatigue and anaemia because the folic acid works with iron, magnesium and zinc to build red blood cells.

✱ storing and serving Because of its fat content, wheatgerm needs to be stored in the refrigerator. Use in baking, on yogurt, breakfast cereal or in drinks.

wheatgerm, pineapple and banana booster

1 Toast **2 tablespoons wheatgerm** and **1 tablespoon sesame seeds** under a grill, stirring a couple of times until the sesame seeds have begun to turn golden. Remove from the grill and leave to cool.

2 Roughly slice **2 bananas** and blend to a rough purée with **75 g (3 oz) pineapple pieces**.

3 Add **450 ml (¾ pint) apple juice** and blend to a fairly smooth juice. Add **300 g (10 oz) natural yogurt** and the cooked wheatgerm and sesame seeds, blend again and serve. **serves 4**

NUTRITIONAL CONTENT PER 100 G RAW: energy 357 kcals | **protein** 27 g | **carbohydrates** 45 g | **fat** 9 g | **fibre** 16 g | **vitamin E** 22 mg | **magnesium** 270 mg | **iron** 8.5 mg | **zinc** 17 mg

211

chickpeas

Also known as garbanzo beans and ceci, chickpeas were cultivated as long ago as 4000 BC. They are a good source of protein and fibre, as well as **energy-producing iron** and manganese.

Like all legumes, chickpeas are ideal for diabetics because the fibre prevents blood sugar levels rising too quickly after a meal. The fibre is great for the digestive system, too, helping prevent constipation, diverticulosis and irritable bowel syndrome (IBS). It may also reduce the risk of bowel cancer.

The soluble fibre in chickpeas, together with magnesium and **folic acid**, offers protection against heart disease.

In addition, chickpeas are a good source of molybdenum, a detoxifying trace mineral that helps rid the body of sulphites. These are commonly used food preservatives, to which some people are particularly sensitive.

✱ storing and serving Store dried chickpeas in an airtight container for up to a year. Once cooked, they can be kept in the refrigerator for a few days or frozen. Add to salads and dips, curries and soups.

spiced chickpea salad

1 Finely chop **1 red onion**, then heat **1 tablespoon olive oil** in a heavy-based saucepan and cook the onion for 5 minutes or until softened.

2 Add **1 teaspoon ground turmeric** and **2 teaspoons cumin seeds** and cook, stirring, for 1–2 minutes. Skin and roughly chop **300g (10 oz) tomatoes** and drain and rinse **400 g (13 oz) canned chickpeas** and add them to the pan with **2 teaspoons lemon juice** and **salt and pepper**. Cook for a further 2–3 minutes.

3 Stir in **2 tablespoons chopped fresh coriander**. **serves 2**

NUTRITIONAL CONTENT PER 100 G CANNED, DRAINED WEIGHT: energy 115 kcals | protein 7 g | carbohydrates 16 g | fat 3 g | fibre 4 g | vitamin E 1.55 mg | calcium 43 mcg | iron 1.5 mg

214

NUTRITIONAL CONTENT PER 100 G BOILED GREEN/BROWN LENTILS:

energy 105 kcals | **protein** 9 g | **carbohydrates** 17 g | **fat** 1 g | **fibre** 4 g | **folate** 30 mcg | **iron** 3.5 mg

lentils

The seeds of a leguminous plant, lentils come in various colours and sizes. Among vegetables, they are second only to soya beans for protein content and so an excellent option for vegetarians, but they need to be eaten with a complementary protein, such as grains.

Because they are high in fibre, lentils keep you feeling full for longer, which makes them useful for slimmers, especially as they are low in fat, and they provide slow-burning energy to keep you going (which also makes them ideal for diabetics). The cholesterol-lowering fibre also means that lentils are excellent for the heart as well as the digestive system.

Lentils contain a good range of nutrients (green and brown lentils even more so than red ones). These include **iron**, useful for those prone to anaemia, some good minerals for bone health and a number of B vitamins, which help to stabilize blood pressure.

Lentils have **anti-inflammatory** properties so are a good food for people with rheumatoid arthritis.

✱ storing and serving Most well-known brands of lentils are ready to use, but some brands need thorough rinsing and picking over to remove dust and grit, before soaking and cooking. Canned lentils are convenient but not quite as nutritious as dried ones.

dhal

1 Briefly fry **6 cloves, 6 cardamoms** and **2.5 cm (1 inch) cinnamon stick** in **4 tablespoons olive oil**.

2 Chop **1 onion** and fry until translucent. Next, finely chop **1 green chilli**, and chop **2.5 cm (1 inch) fresh ginger** and **1 garlic clove.** Add them all to the pan with **½ teaspoon garam masala**. Cook for 5 minutes.

3 Stir in **250 g (8 oz) lentils** and fry for 1 minute. Add **salt** and sufficient water to come about 3 cm (1¼ inches) above the lentils. Bring to the boil, cover and simmer for 20 minutes. Sprinkle over **4 tablespoons lemon juice**, stir and serve. **serves 4**

beans

Beans, lentils and chickpeas are all pulses with very similar health-boosting properties. A **low-fat, filling protein food** with slow-release sugars, beans are particularly good for the digestive system. One study even suggests that a serving of beans four times a week may **reduce the risk of heart disease** by 22 per cent.

Beans, usually available dried, are edible seeds. They are highly nutritious, resulting in the expression to be **'full of beans'**, meaning to be lively. Dried beans, such as aduki, mung and soya beans, can be sprouted, which makes them rich in both B and C vitamins.

Beans also contain phyto-oestrogens, which can help tackle erratic periods and premenstrual syndrome (PMS) and relieve some menopausal symptoms.

Beans contain lignans and isoflavones, which help prevent hormone-dependent cancers.

✱ storing and serving Store dried beans in airtight containers in the cupboard. Cook them to serve as a simple side dish or use them in thick soups, stews and casseroles. Mash them for use in dips and pâtés or add them to salads.

cannellini bean and sun-dried tomato salad

1 Heat **2 tablespoons olive oil** in a frying pan. Add **1 crushed garlic clove** and sauté until golden. Remove from pan.

2 Drain and rinse **425 g (14 oz) can cannellini beans**, place in a mixing bowl and stir in the garlic. Add **1 sliced red onion, 125 g (4 oz) chopped sun-dried tomatoes (drained from their oil), 1 tablespoon chopped black olives, 2 teaspoons chopped capers, 2 teaspoons chopped thyme, 1 tablespoon parsley leaves, 1 tablespoon extra virgin olive oil, 1 tablespoon lemon juice, salt and pepper** and mix well. **serves 4**

NUTRITIONAL CONTENT PER 100 G CANNELLINI BEANS, CANNED : energy 94 kcals | **protein** 7 g | **carbohydrates** 14 g | **fat** 0 g | **fibre** 6 g | **calcium** 65 mg | **iron** 2.5 mg | **potassium** 320 mg

217

chillies

Chilli peppers, which come in a range of sizes, shapes, colours and heat levels, contain the antioxidant vitamins A (beta-carotene), C and E, plus **folic acid** and **potassium**. They are, therefore, good for general health and for protecting the heart.

Countless healing properties have been attributed to chillies, but many claims have yet to be validated. What is known is that capsaicin, which accounts for the 'heat' of chillies, can help prevent dangerous blood clots and help with weight loss, as capsaicin both suppresses the appetite and helps to boost metabolism.

The World Health Organization (WHO) has reported a link between capsaicin-rich diets and reduced death rates from cancer.

Research from Australia shows chillies have an effect on insulin so are good for regulating blood sugar levels.

✱ **storing and serving** Keep fresh chillies in the refrigerator, and dried chillies and chilli powder in airtight jars, away from the heat and light of cooking. Removing the seeds and membranes of fresh chillies will minimize their heat but will also remove the health-boosting capsaicin.

NUTRITIONAL CONTENT PER 100 G RAW: energy 20 kcals | protein 3 g | carbohydrates 1 g | fat 1 g | fibre 2 g | vitamin C 120 mg | carotene 175 mcg | folate 29 mcg | potassium 220 mg

fresh chilli chutney

1 Purée **250 g (8 oz) fresh green chillies** with **250 ml (8 fl oz) vinegar** and transfer to a hot, dry sterilized jar.

2 Top up with vinegar to prevent a mould from forming and tightly cover the jar, The chutney will change from bright to dark green in colour about 1–2 weeks but will keep indefinitely. **makes about 250 g (8 oz)**

220

ginger

Ginger is a centuries-old digestive aid and a popular remedy for nausea, particularly travel sickness and morning sickness. It can also help relieve indigestion and heartburn, and is useful for treating coughs, colds and flu-like symptoms.

The health-boosting properties of ginger appear to be due to its powerful gingerols. These act as **anti-inflammatory** agents, so ginger can reduce the pain and swelling of rheumatism and arthritis and may help alleviate asthma, painful periods and migraines.

The gingerol compounds appear to be antioxidants, and initial studies suggest that they may provide some protection against cancer. Similarly, ginger is believed by some to lower cholesterol and protect against heart disease, but more research is required.

Ginger boosts the metabolism, so slimmers may find it useful for accelerating calorie burning.

✱ storing and serving Fresh unpeeled ginger root will keep for up to two weeks in the refrigerator and up to six months if frozen. Use fresh ginger in curries, stir-fries, salad dressings and lemonade.

spring onion and ginger rice

1 Wash **300 g (10 oz) long grain rice**. Transfer to a pan with **1 teaspoon salt, 3 bruised cardamom pods** and **600 ml (1 pint) water**. Simmer over a low heat for 5 minutes. Cover tightly and cook for 5 minutes until tender.

2 Deseed and chop **1 green chilli**, crush **2 garlic cloves**, thinly slice **2 courgettes** and chop a **bunch of spring onions**. Stir-fry in **2 tablespoons olive oil** with **1 tablespoon grated fresh ginger** for 1 minute. Add the rice, **2 tablespoons chopped fresh coriander, 2 tablespoons light soy sauce** and **1 tablespoon lemon juice.** Stir over a low heat for 2 minutes. **serves 4**

NUTRITIONAL CONTENT PER 100 G ROOT, RAW: energy 38 kcals I **protein** 1 g I **carbohydrates** 7 g I **fat** 1 g I **fibre** 2 g I **vitamin C** 4 mg I **potassium** 320 mg I **magnesium** 35 mg

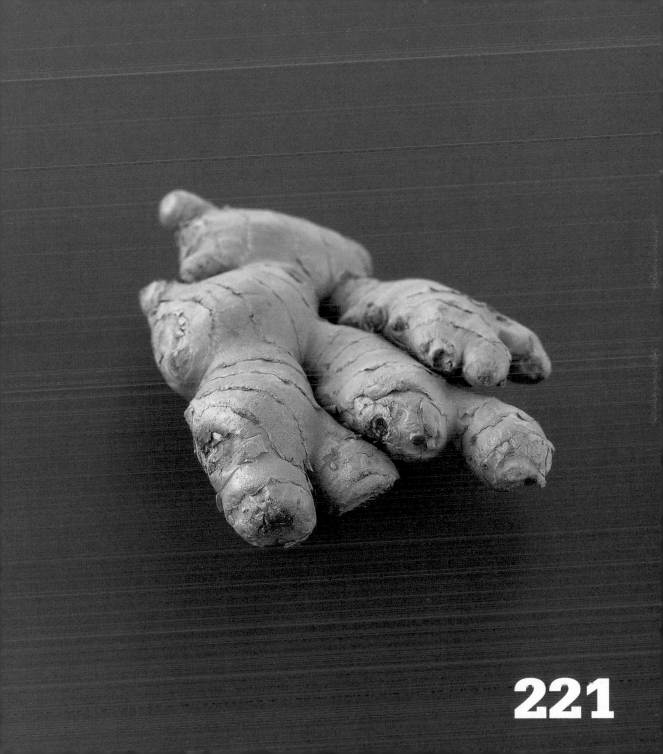

221

garlic

Cultivated as early as 2000 BC in Mesopotamia and Egypt, garlic was believed by the ancient Greeks and Romans to possess magical properties.

Garlic contains powerful sulphurous compounds thought to slow or prevent the growth of cancer and to **stimulate the liver's detoxification function**. The same compounds, plus vitamins B_6 and C and manganese and **selenium**, make garlic highly protective towards the heart. Eating garlic regularly can help keep arteries clear and lower high cholesterol levels; it also reduces the risk of blood clotting and reduces high blood pressure.

Garlic is a natural antibiotic and, taken regularly, can build up resistance to infection. It is a decongestant, helping to relieve the symptoms of colds, coughs and flu. It is also an **anti-inflammatory**, and may help protect against asthma and rheumatoid arthritis.

✱ storing and serving Store fresh garlic in an uncovered container away from heat and sunlight. An unbroken bulb will keep for a couple of months. Eating a clove a day is recommended by health experts – try chewing parsley or coffee beans to counteract the smell.

garlic and almond soup

1 Tear **50 g (2 oz) bread** into small pieces, put in a bowl and cover with water. In another bowl cover **125 g (4 oz) raisins** with water. Leave to soak for 30–60 minutes.

2 Remove the bread from the water and squeeze dry. Blend to a smooth paste with **125 g (4 oz) toasted blanched almonds**.

3 Add **3 tablespoons olive oil**, **3 crushed garlic cloves**, the raisins and **900 ml (1½ pints) milk** (or water). Blend to make a smooth soup. Chill for 2–3 hours before serving in small bowls. **serves 6**

NUTRITIONAL CONTENT PER 100 G RAW: energy 98 kcals | **protein** 8 g | **carbohydrates** 16 g | **fat** 1 g | **fibre** 4 g | **vitamin B_6** 0.38 mg | **potasssium** 620 mg | **manganese** 0.5 mg | **selenium** 2 mcg

fresh herbs

A recent study by the US Department of Agriculture found thyme, rosemary, sage, peppermint and particularly oregano, also known as wild marjoram, to be **highly antioxidant**. In fact, oregano has four times more free radical-fighting antioxidants than blueberries.

Rosemary can help **boost the immune system**. It is especially useful at exam time because it increases blood flow to the brain, improving concentration. The menthol in peppermint stops muscle spasm so helps treat indigestion, heartburn, flatulence and nausea.

Basil and sage are **anti-inflammatories**. Both can help relieve the symptoms of rheumatoid arthritis, asthma and inflammatory bowel conditions. Basil and thyme have antibacterial qualities, and adding either to salad dressings can help remove a diarrhoea-causing bacteria from salad leaves. Parsley helps kidney function, relieves gout and combats anaemia.

✱ storing and serving Fresh herbs are more health-boosting than dried ones, so substitute one tablespoon chopped fresh herb for 1 teaspoon of the dried equivalent whenever possible in cooking. Fresh herbs freeze well if you have a surplus.

herby risotto

1 Finely chop **1 onion** and **1 garlic clove** and sauté in **50 g (2 oz) butter** with **2 tablespoons olive oil** for 5 minutes.

2 Add **300 g (10 oz) Arborio rice** and stir well to coat the grains with butter and oil. Add **1 litre (1¾ pints) hot vegetable stock**, a ladleful at a time, stirring until each addition is absorbed. Continue adding stock, cooking until the rice is creamy but the grains are still firm.

3 Mix in handful each of chopped **parsley**, **basil**, **oregano** and **thyme**, **75 g (3 oz) butter** and **125 g (4 oz) grated Toma cheese**. Season with **salt and pepper** and stir well. Cover and leave to rest for a few minutes before serving, **serves 4**

NUTRITIONAL CONTENT PER 100 G FRESH BASIL (OREGANO): energy 40 (66) kcals | **protein** 3 (2) g | **carbohydrates** 5 (10) g | **fat** 1 (2) g | **fibre** 0 (0) g | **potassium** 300 (330) mg

226

horseradish

Thanks to its strong volatile oils, which are similar to those found in mustard, horseradish has an intensity of flavour strong enough to bring tears to the eyes.

Its pungency explains why horseradish can relieve cold symptoms and congested sinuses by dissolving mucus. It can also relieve water retention, or bloating, and may provide some relief from rheumatism.

Its **antibiotic properties** mean horseradish can fight infections such as tonsillitis and protect the gut from bacteria, including listeria and *E. coli*.

Horseradish is a member of the brassica family and contains the phytochemicals called **glucosinolates**, which have been shown to fight cancer by suppressing tumour growths. Glucosinolates also increase the liver's ability to detoxify.

✻ storing and serving Horseradish is most commonly available as horseradish sauce or as prepared horseradish, which is made from shredded and pounded horseradish mixed with vinegar. Creamed horseradish is a creamier version. Once opened, store prepared and creamed horseradish in the refrigerator for up to six months. Traditionally paired with roast beef, horseradish also goes well with smoked salmon and adds a zing to mashed potato, cream cheese or mayonnaise.

horseradish mash

1 Peel and dice **750 g (1½ lb) potatoes** and cook in boiling water for about 20 minutes or until tender. Drain well and return to the pan.

2 Add **50 g (2 oz) butter, 150 ml (¼ pint) single cream** and **2–3 tablespoons freshly grated horseradish** and mash well. Season with **salt and pepper** and serve. **serves 4**

chicken and turkey

As long as you avoid eating the skin, chicken and turkey are healthy alternatives to red meat.

If you have trouble sleeping try eating poultry in the evening. Both chicken and turkey are rich in an amino acid called tryptophan, which helps regulate sleep. Tryptophan can also lift the spirits and the **zinc** in turkey can assist in combating depression and anxiety.

Eating poultry may help prevent cancer, because chicken and, to a lesser extent, turkey are good sources of two **anti-cancer** nutrients, **niacin** and **selenium**.

Chicken, which is a good source of the B vitamins required by the brain for memory maintenance, is also good for preventing forgetfulness and age-related mental decline. Indeed, its vitamin B_3 (niacin) content may help protect against Alzheimer's disease.

✱ **storing and serving** Keep raw poultry closely wrapped in the refrigerator to avoid contaminating other foods, and wash your hands and utensils well after handling it. To avoid the risk of infection, chicken and turkey should always be cooked right through until no pink meat is left and any juices run clear.

chicken with rosemary and garlic

1 Mix together **2 tablespoons olive oil**, **2 tablespoons white wine vinegar**, **2 tablespoons chopped rosemary**, **3 crushed garlic cloves**, **1 teaspoon paprika** and the pared rind of **1 lemon** and season with **salt and pepper. Add 4 skinless chicken fillets** (cut in to long thin strips) and mix well. Leave to marinate for 10 minutes.

2 Cook the chicken and the marinade over a moderate heat, stirring constantly, for 15 minutes.

3 Stir in a **handful of chopped flat leaf parsley** immediately before serving. **serves 4**

NUTRITIONAL CONTENT PER 100 G RAW BREAST CHICKEN (TURKEY): energy 116 (103) kcals | **protein** 22 (23) g | **carbohydrates** 0 (0) g | **fat 3** (1) g | **fibre** 0 (0) g | **zinc** 0.7 (1.2) mg

229

game fowl

Traditionally hunted in the wild, game birds are now often commercially reared. Because they forage for their food, they are more active and therefore leaner than domestic birds. Their fat is mainly monounsaturated.

Guinea fowl meat is a good source of heart-protective vitamin B_6 and of two **anti-cancer** nutrients, **selenium** and **niacin**.

Pheasant and partridge are excellent sources of **iron**, partridge providing about three times as much as beef. Lack of iron can cause anaemia and reduced concentration. Pheasant and partridge also provide **phosphorus** and **calcium**, essential for the formation of strong bones; **potassium**, which helps prevent high blood pressure; and vitamin B_6 and **folic acid**, both of which help reduce excess levels of homocysteine, a risk factor for heart attacks.

Partridge contains high levels of sulphur, the 'beauty mineral', essential for glossy hair, skin and nails.

✱ storing and serving Game birds can easily dry out, so require basting while roasting. Older birds are tougher and are best casseroled slowly.

grilled guinea fowl

1 Put **4 boneless guinea fowl breasts** on a lightly oiled grill pan, brush with **olive oil** and season with **salt and pepper**. Place the pan under a preheated hot grill and cook for 10 minutes on each side.

2 Blend **3 crushed garlic cloves**, **4 chopped anchovy fillets**, a large **handful of flat leaf parsley**, a handful each of **rocket**, **sorrel** and **basil** leaves and **2 tablespoons lemon juice**. With the motor running, slowly drizzle in **125 ml (4 fl oz) olive oil**. Season and blend again.

3 Serve the guinea fowl with the herb sauce. **serves 4**

NUTRITIONAL CONTENT PER 100 G RAW GUINEA FOWL (ROAST PHEASANT):
energy 110 (213) kcals | **protein** 21 (32) g | **carbohydrates** 0 (0) g | **fat** 3 (9) g | **fibre** 0 (0) g

231

lean red meat

In contrast to greasy hamburgers, big steaks dripping with fat and roast pork with crispy crackling, lean beef, lamb or pork eaten in moderation can actually boost your health. It is a good source of protein, **zinc**, **selenium** and **iron**, plus vitamins B_3 (**niacin**), B_6 and B_{12}, which can all help keep the heart in good shape.

B vitamins are heart protective because they reduce excess levels of an amino acid called homocysteine, which can cause strokes and heart attacks. Vitamin B_3 (niacin), B_{12} and selenium are all linked with a reduced risk of cancer, particularly bowel cancer.

Eating lean meat can **boost the immune system** thanks to the high levels of **zinc**, which is important for sexual health, prostate health and wound healing.

✱ **choosing lean meat** Opt for the leanest cuts of meat (those from the animal's legs) and always remove all visible fat. Pork is often regarded as a fatty meat, but pork escalopes actually have less saturated fat than beef or lamb and are almost on a par with chicken for their fat content. Buy organic meat to avoid the residues of growth hormones and antibiotics found in non-organic meat.

green peppercorn steak

1 Cook **4 x 75 g (3 oz) fillet steaks** for 2–3 minutes on each side on a preheated hot griddle pan. Remove from the pan and keep hot.

2 Add **1 tablespoon green peppercorns** in brine, drained, **2 tablespoons light soy sauce**, **1 teaspoon balsamic vinegar** and **8 halved cherry tomatoes** to the griddle pan. Allow the liquids to sizzle for 2 minutes or until the tomatoes are soft.

3 Spoon the sauce over the steaks and garnish with **thyme sprigs**. **serves 4**

NUTRITIONAL CONTENT PER 100 G LEAN RAW BEEF: energy 123 kcals I **protein** 17 g I **carbohydrates** 0 g I **fat** 5 g I **fibre** 0 g I **folate** 10 mcg I **iron** 2.1 mg I **zinc** 4.3 mg I **selenium** 3 mcg

233

NUTRITIONAL CONTENT PER 100 G RAW: energy 103 kcals | protein 22 g | carbohydrates 0 g | fat 2 g | fibre 0 g | potassium 340 mg | iron 3.3 mg | selenium 9 mcg | zinc 2.4 mg

venison

Iron-rich venison is the healthiest of the red meats, containing less than half the saturated fat of lean beef. In fact, venison's **low-calorie**, **low-fat** and **high-protein** profile is similar to that of chicken and salmon. Venison is also a surprising source of essential **omega-3 fatty acids**. These 'good' fats reduce the risk factors (high cholesterol levels and blood clots) for stroke and heart attacks. They also support brain health and development and can help deal with depression.

A source of **iron**, venison is good for those prone to fatigue and anaemia and in need of an iron boost.

Venison also provides a number of B vitamins, which are important for producing energy. Two of these, vitamins B_6 and B_{12}, have cardio-protective properties, and vitamin B_{12} may help protect against osteoporosis and bowel cancer.

✱ **storing and serving** Venison is available as whole joints, steaks, chops or minced meat. Store it according to whether it is fresh or frozen. You can substitute venison for beef in virtually any recipe. Use it in hearty casseroles, pasta dishes or in kebabs for the barbecue. Overcooking it will toughen it.

griddled venison steaks with red fruit sauce

1 Mix together **1 teaspoon crushed juniper berries** and a **pinch of pepper** and spread over both sides of **4 x 175 g (6 oz) venison steaks** (fillet or loin). Leave overnight.

2 Put **125 g (4 oz) redcurrant jelly**, **125 g (4 oz) cranberries**, the grated rind and juice of **1 orange** and **2 tablespoons red wine** in a small saucepan. Simmer gently for 10 minutes, stirring constantly.

3 Griddle the venison steaks for 3 minutes on each side for rare or 5 minutes for well done. Serve with the sauce and garnish with **shredded orange rind**. **serves 4**

235

NUTRITIONAL CONTENT PER 100 G RAW LAMB (CALF): energy 179 (153) kcals | protein 20 (20) g | carbohydrates 2 (2) g | fat 10 (7) g | fibre 0 (0) g | folate 220 (240) g | iron 9 (8) mg

liver

Liver is well known for being a rich source of **iron**, which helps prevent or cure anaemia. It also contains vitamins B_1, B_2, B_6 and B_{12}, which are necessary for the formation of haemoglobin and for brain function.

Because the vitamin A levels in farmed liver are very high, pregnant women should not eat liver or liver products because it could harm the developing foetus. However, both foods are recommended after the birth, especially for breastfeeding mothers.

Eating liver may provide some protection against heart disease and cancer because it is an excellent source of the cardio-protective vitamin B_{12} and **folic acid**, as well as the antioxidant minerals **zinc**, **selenium** and copper, which protect against damaging free radicals and may prevent prostate cancer.

Although liver contains more fat than lean meat, most of this is in the form of polyunsaturated fats, so it is not harmful and is unlikely to raise blood cholesterol levels.

✱ **buying organic** Because the liver is the organ responsible for filtering toxins, toxic substances are likely to collect here. It therefore makes sense to eat only liver from an organically reared animal to avoid consuming pesticides or other chemical residues.

quick liver one-pot

1 Thinly slice **2 onions** and **3 carrots** and cook in **1 tablespoon olive oil** with **4 rashers of lean back bacon** over a low heat for 10 minutes.

2 Add **1 tablespoon redcurrant jelly** and **1 tablespoon tomato purée** and cook for a further 2 minutes, stirring occasionally.

3 Add **500 g (1 lb) lamb's liver**, cover and leave to cook for about 5 minutes. Stir, season with **salt and pepper**, re-cover and cook for a further 2–3 minutes. Serve immediately, with mashed potatoes and a selection of green vegetables. **serves 4**

tea

The subject of a great deal of research, tea offers powerful antioxidant properties. Black, oolong and green teas all come from the same plant, but their leaves are processed differently.

The least processed of the three, green tea, is the most beneficial. Its main health-boosting ingredients are tannins and catechins, antioxidants with effective cancer-prevention and heart-protective properties.

Numerous studies have shown that green tea-drinking populations have a reduced risk of a huge range of disorders and diseases. Besides combating cancer and heart disease, drinking green tea can lower blood sugar levels and help prevent type 2 (late-onset) diabetes. It may have some effect on the AIDS virus, and it can help prevent osteoporosis.

Green tea is useful for treating diarrhoea and for killing the bacteria responsible for the stomach upset.

Both green and black teas help combat the flu virus.

✱ **storing and serving** Keep tea in a cupboard, not a refrigerator. Use boiling water for black and oolong tea, but use slightly cooler water for green tea.

Earl Grey brûlée

1 Bring **600 ml (1 pint) single cream** to the boil. Stir in **8 teaspoons Earl Grey tea leaves**. Stand for 15 minutes.

2 Beat together **8 egg yolks** and **125 g (4 oz) caster sugar**. Reheat the tea-flavoured cream and stir it into the egg mixture bit by bit.

3 Strain the custard into 6 ramekins in a roasting pan. Pour warm water into the pan to come halfway up the sides of the dishes and bake in a preheated oven, 180°C (350°F), Gas Mark 4, for 20–25 minutes.

4 Leave to cool then chill for 3–4 hours. Before serving, sprinkle the tops with **50 g (2 oz) caster sugar**. Caramelize with a blowtorch, and serve at room temperature. **serves 6**

NUTRITIONAL CONTENT PER 100 ML INFUSED, BLACK/GREEN: energy 0 kcals | **protein** 0.1 g | **carbohydrates** 0 g | **fat** 0 g | **fibre** 0 g | **potassium** 17 mg (analysis done using distilled water – mineral content will vary according to local water used)

239

glossary

glossary

Absorption Process by which nutrients are taken from the intestine into the bloodstream and into cells.

ACE vitamins Vitamins A, C and E, which are especially renowned for their strong antioxidant powers.

Additives The term commonly used to refer to synthetic colourings or preservatives, often added to processed food to enhance the appearance and shelf life of the final product.

Allicin A beneficial sulphurous compound found in garlic that dilates blood vessels, thereby reducing the risk of blood clots and helping protect the heart.

Alpha-carotene A type of carotenoid found in carrots and other vegetables. A powerful antioxidant, it helps protect cells from the damage inflicted by free radicals and, like beta-carotene, can be converted in the body to vitamin A.

Alpha-linolenic acid An omega-3 essential fatty acid, vital for the body's health.

Alzheimer's disease A disease that kills brain cells, causing progressive memory loss and dementia. Drug treatment appears to slow progression of the disease but there is currently no cure.

Amino acids The 20 different building blocks of proteins. Some of them, for example asparagine and glutamine, can be synthesized in our bodies. The others (known as the essential amino acids) have to be obtained from protein foods in the diet, such as meat, fish, beans, and lentils. Essential amino acids include leucine, tryptophan, lysine and tyrosine.

Anaemia A condition in which the blood's oxygen-carrying capacity is lessened. Anaemia is caused by various conditions, including excessive menstrual bleeding and lack of iron, vitamin B12 or folic acid in the diet. The symptoms include pallor, weakness and fatigue, depression and low resistance to infections.

Anthocyanidins A group of flavonoids found in red, purple and blue fruits and vegetables.

Antibacterial The ability to kill bacteria, but not viruses.

Antibodies Proteins produced by the immune system in response to 'foreign' invaders (antigens), for example those belonging to viruses.

Following exposure to a particular infection, the body 'remembers' the foreign protein and can figh off the infection more quickly next time, .

Anti-inflammatory
The ability to reduce inflammation.

Antimicrobial The ability to kill both bacteria and viruses.

Antioxidants Beneficial natural substances found in foods that rid the body of the damaging free radicals that cause oxidation, resulting in better general health and delayed ageing.

Antiseptic The ability to prevent the growth or spread of micro-organisms, inhibiting their action but not killing them.

Antiviral The ability to kill viruses, but not bacteria.

Ascorbic acid Vitamin C.

Asparagine *See* Amino acids.

Atherosclerosis A build-up of fatty deposits (atheroma) within artery walls — a risk factor for heart disease, heart attack and stroke.

Beta-carotene An antioxidant nutrient found in dark green, red, orange and yellow fruits and vegetables, which is converted in the body to vitamin A.

Bile A bitter fluid produced by the liver, stored in the gall bladder and released when required by the digestive process to break down fats and absorb vitamins.

Bioavailability The degree to which a substance, for example a nutrient, is absorbed or becomes available to the body.

Biotin One of the B vitamins involved in the body's production of energy.

Blood sugar Refers to levels of sugar (glucose) in the blood, formed from digesting food and which the body uses for energy. Blood sugar levels are affected by the type of food consumed. High blood sugar levels are typical of people with diabetes.

Bowel The intestine, especially referring to the large intestine, concerned with the digestion and absorption of food.

Brassicas A family of edible plants, also called cruciferous vegetables, believed to provide protection against various cancers. Broccoli, cabbage, cauliflower, kale, brussels sprouts and radishes are all brassicas.

Bromelain An enzyme found in pineapple, which is effective in treating blood clots, the cause of thrombosis.

Caffeine A naturally occurring and mildly addictive substance found in tea, coffee, cocoa and cola drinks, which stimulates the central nervous system and heart, and is a diuretic. Caffeine increases alertness although, in excessive amounts, it can cause insomnia.

Calciferol Vitamin D.

Calories Strictly speaking kilocalories (abbreviated to kcal), these are units of energy values of foods.

Cancer Disease involving abnormal or uncontrolled growth of cells that can occur in any organ of the body.

Capsaicin An active compound in capsicum peppers and chillies.

Carbohydrate A major class of food comprising the sugars and starches found in grains and grain products (e.g. breads, rice), plus fruits and vegetables. Once digested, these turn into glucose, which is stored in the liver until required for energy.

Carcinogen Any cancer-triggering substance.

Cardiovascular disease
See Heart disease.

Carotenoid A group of powerful antioxidants, including alpha- and beta-carotene, responsible for the pigment of dark green, yellow, orange and red fruits and vegetables. Many of the carotenoids convert to vitamin A in the body.

Chlorophyll The green pigment found in plants that traps the energy of the sun for photosynthesis.

Cholesterol A fat-like substance made by the body and carried in the blood. When blood cholesterol levels are too high, cholesterol may be deposited on the insides of blood vessels, thereby narrowing them and causing blockages, resulting in heart disease. There are two types of cholesterol – high-density lipoprotein (HDL), which is beneficial because it reduces blood cholesterol, and low-density lipoprotein (LDL), which `is dangerous as it encourages cholesterol deposits in blood vessels.

Cobalamine Vitamin B12, involved in the production of red blood cells and nerve cells.

Collagen Elastic protein that forms connective tissue in the body, for example tendon, cartilage and bone.

Colon The lower and largest part of the intestine, or bowel.

Cruciferous vegetables
See Brassicas.

Degenerative condition
A serious ailment that get worse with time.

Detoxification The process of removing toxins from the body, a build-up of which can contribute to ill health. The results of detoxifying include clearer skin, more regular bowel movements and more efficient kidney and liver function.

Diabetes A disease caused by the body's inability to produce or properly use insulin, the hormone needed to convert sugar and other foods into energy. Diabetes complications include heart disease, blindness and kidney disease. Diabetes can often be managed through lifestyle changes, including diet, and medication.

Diuretic A substance that causes an increase in urine production, dehydrating the body.

DNA Deoxyribonucleic acid, the genetic material in the body's cells that carries information on cell growth, division and function.

Dopamine A chemical found in the brain that is an important neurotransmitter.

Ellagic acid A flavonoid believed to deplete cancer-causing substances in the body.

Empty calories A term used for food such as alcohol and refined sugar, which contain calories but no nutrients.

Enzyme Protein substances involved in every chemical reaction in the body, for example digestive enzymes are responsible for the digestion and absorption of food into the body.

Fats Vital in the diet for maintaining healthy skin and hair, regulating cholesterol, absorbing fat-soluble vitamins, promoting healthy cell function and providing energy. Fats are generally classified as saturated, monounsaturated or polyunsaturated. The food we eat contains varying proportions of these fats.

Fibre, dietary The indigestible parts of plant foods, which pass through the digestive system, absorbing water and accelerating elimination of waste. Fibre helps keep the digestive system healthy, and regulates cholesterol and blood sugar levels, reducing the risk of bowel cancer, heart disease and diabetes.

Flavonoids/bioflavonoids A group of antioxidant plant pigments, including flavones and flavanones, which work in synergy with vitamin C, neutralizing free radicals and helping reduce the risk of cancer.

Folate A B vitamin, also known as folic acid, required for the formation of red blood cells and for supporting the nervous system. A deficiency of folate in a woman before conceiving or during early pregnancy can cause anaemia in the mum-to-be and neural tube defects in the baby. Folate also helps protect the heart by preventing build-up of homocysteine.

Folic acid *See* Folate.

Fortified foods Foods that have had nutrients added to them to benefit health, for example bread fortified with selenium and breakfast cereals fortified with calcium and folic acid.

Free radicals Abnormal, electrochemically imbalanced molecules produced by the body as a natural waste product. They can set off a damaging chain reaction of oxidation within the body, resulting in wrinkles, sagging skin, age spots and the onset of age-related diseases. The damage may be repaired by antioxidants.

Functional foods Foods with health-promoting or disease-preventing properties and for which a health claim has been authorized.

Gastrointestinal The complete digestive system.

Glucose The major sugar in the body and a key energy provider.

Glucosinolates Sulphurous organic compounds, for example sulphoraphane, found in brassicas and believed to help prevent a variety of cancers.

Glutamine *See* Amino acids.

Glutathione Water-soluble antioxidant found in the body, which can destroy toxins such as carcinogens.

Glycaemic index A ranking system rating the effect of different carbohydrate-rich foods on blood sugar levels two hours after consumption. Foods with a low GI release glucose slowly into the bloodstream, which is better for energy provision and blood sugar levels.

Haemoglobin The iron-containing protein molecule in red blood cells, responsible for the red colour of blood.

Heart attack Any sudden severe instance of abnormal heart functioning often caused by a sudden decrease in blood supply to the heart and resulting in chest pain.

Heart disease Also known as cardiovascular disease, this covers a range of problems affecting the heart and blood vessels, including atherosclerosis, coronary artery disease, angina, heart failure and high blood pressure.

Herperidin A flavonoid, also known as hesperidin, found in citrus fruits.

High blood pressure
Blood pressure is the force of blood against artery walls. High blood pressure, also known as hypertension, is a condition in which arterial blood pressure is persistently raised, It can lead to strokes, heart attacks, heart disease and kidney failure. Diet plays a large role in both preventing and managing the condition.

Homocysteine An amino acid normally found in the blood. Raised levels of homocysteine are associated with an increased risk of heart disease. Folic acid can help lower raised homocysteine levels.

Hormones Chemical messengers produced and released within the body in tiny amounts and which circulate in the bloodstream. Imbalances can cause conditions like diabetes.

Hydrogenation The chemical process of turning unsaturated liquid fat (vegetable oil) into solid or semi-solid fat (margarine).

Hypertension
See High blood pressure.

Hypotension Abnormally low blood pressure.

Immune system The body's defence system, composed mainly of antibodies and white blood cells, which works to resist infection.

Insulin A hormone used to store glucose (sugar) and help regulate its concentration in the blood. Diabetics either can't produce adequate amounts of insulin or they can't use it efficiently and therefore have abnormal blood sugar levels.

Isoflavones A type of phyto-oestrogen found in soya beans and soya products, which may reduce symptoms relating to the menopause and may be useful for treating cancer.

Isothiocyanates Beneficial phytonutrients responsible for the intense 'heat' in plants such as horseradish, radishes and mustards.

Kaempferol A flavonoid found in almonds, cranberries, strawberries and peas.

Kidney stones Deposits of calcium salts in the kidneys that can cause pain and infection.

Lactobacillus *See* Probiotics.

Leucine *See* Amino acids.

Lignans Type of phyto-oestrogen found in flaxseed, wholegrains and various fruits and vegetables, which may lower cholesterol, thereby protecting against heart disease and some cancers.

Linoleic acid An omega-6 essential fatty acid, vital for the body's health. Along with alpha-linoleic acid, one of the two main dietary polyunsaturated fatty acids.

Lutein A type of carotenoid which, like zeaxanthin, promotes healthy eyes, reducing the risk of cataracts and age-related macular degeneration.

Lycopene A carotenoid which reduces the risk of cancer, heart disease and age-related eye problems. It is found in red fruit and vegetables and is particularly available in processed tomato products, such as canned tomatoes and tomato purée.

Lysine *See* Amino acids.

Macular degeneration Progressively poor vision due to degenerating blood supply to the retina. A common cause of blindness in the elderly.

Melatonin A hormone produced in the brain's pineal gland involved in regulating sleep and maintaining the body's natural time clock.

Metabolism All the biochemical processes that occur within the body by which it survives, grows, produces energy and eliminates waste, for example breathing, blood circulation and digestion.

Minerals Inorganic elements essential for normal body function and good health. Some minerals are essential components in the body, for example calcium in bones and iron in the blood's haemoglobin. Others help regulate metabolic processes.

Monounsaturated fat Fatty acids found in nuts, avocados and olive oil, which help maintain healthy cholesterol levels and are therefore thought to protect against heart disease.

Naringin A bitter-tasting flavonoid compound.

Nervous system The body's network of specialized cells, including the brain, which transmit nerve impulses around the body.

Neural tube defects Malformation of the brain or spinal cord (neurological system) during development in the womb. A good intake of folic acid by women before conception and during early pregnancy greatly reduces the risk to the baby.

Neurotransmitters
Biochemical messengers that enable nerves in the brain to communicate.

Niacin Vitamin B3, one of the B vitamins involved in the body's production of energy.

Nitrosamines Carcinogenic chemical compounds found in certain processed foods.

Nutraceuticals
See Functional foods.

Nutrient density Nutrient dense foods provide substantial amounts of vitamins and minerals relative to their calorie content. Calorie-dense foods supply calories yet relatively few nutrients.

Oestrogen Group of hormones present in both men and women, but involved mainly with the female reproductive system.

Omega-3 Essential fatty acids (EFAs) which must be acquired from the diet. Found in oily fish, walnuts and flaxseed, omega-3s help reduce the risk of heart disease, improve mental function and deal with joint pain. Most people need to include more omega-3s in their diets.

Omega-6 Essential fatty acids (EFAs) which must be acquired from the diet, found in corn and sunflower oils, nuts and seeds. Many people in modern industrialized societies are actually consuming too many omega-6 fats (from polyunsaturated margarines and oils, often 'hidden' in manufactured baked goods) at the expense of omega-3s.

ORAC Oxygen Radical Absorbance Capacity, a test developed at the Human Nutrition Research Center on Aging at Tufts University, Boston, US, to determine the antioxidant power of different foods.

Organic foods Organic fruit and vegetables grown without the use of synthetic pesticides, fertilizers or fungicides. Organic meat comes from animals raised without routine antibiotics or growth hormones.

Osteoporosis Skeletal disease caused by loss of bone density. The bones become very fragile and prone to fracture. Osteoporosis is more common in women, especially after the menopause, and often goes undetected until a fracture occurs. A good calcium intake during childhood, adolescence and early adulthood, plus regular weight-bearing exercise can help prevent the disease occurring.

Oxalic acid A substance found in certain foods, for example spinach, which is poisonous in excessive amounts. Anyone with kidney or bladder stones should avoid foods containing oxalic acid because it can aggravate these conditions.

Oxidization Oxidative damage to the cells of the body ('rusting'), due to the action of unstable, unpaired free radicals which take a hydrogen ion from nearby molecules so as to 'pair off'. These newly unpaired molecules then do the same thing, setting up a chain reaction within the body that leads to tissue damage but can be stopped by antioxidants.

Pantothenic acid Vitamin B5, one of the B vitamins involved in the body's production of energy.

Papain An enzyme found in papayas, which helps in the digestion of protein.

Pectin A soluble fibre found in the pith and cellular membranes of many ripe fruits and vegetables. It helps maintain bowel function and lower blood cholesterol levels.

Phytochemicals
See Phytonutrients.

Phyto-oestrogens Substances found in plants which are similar to human oestrogens. They are thought to help reduce some of the symptoms of premenstrual syndrome and the menopause.

Phytonutrients Plant chemicals at the forefront of scientific research into food and health and of interest for their role

in preventing serious diseases such as cancer, heart disease, asthma and arthritis.

Polyunsaturated fat
Fatty acids that are usually liquid at room temperature, for example vegetable oils, and can be converted to trans fats by hydrogenation.

Precursor A biochemical substance, from which another more definitive product is formed.

Proanthocyanidins
Type of tannin found in cranberries, cocoa and chocolate, believed to help improve urinary tract health and reduce the risk of heart disease.

Probiotics Live microorganisms, for example lactobacilli and bifidobacteria, which are added to foods such as yogurt to improve gastrointestinal health.

Protein A complex compound formed from nitrogen and amino acids, which is required in the diet by our bodies for growth and repair. Proteins are found mainly in animal products, as well as in grains and pulses.

Pro-vitamin A substance that can be converted via the body's normal metabolic processes into a vitamin. Carotene, for example, is a pro-vitamin of vitamin A.

Pterostilbene An antioxidant compound found in blueberries and grapes.

Purines Natural substances found in virtually all foods and useful in the body. High-purine foods like offal, anchovies and sardines should be avoided by gout sufferers since purines are broken down into uric acid, an accumulation of which is responsible for gout.

Pyridoxine Vitamin B6, essential for many processes within the body, including the formation of new cells (including red blood and nerve cells), the production of energy and balancing hormonal changes in women.

Quercetin A flavonoid with anti-inflammatory and anti-cancer properties, found in the skins of apples and red onions.

249

RDA Recommended Daily/ Dietary Allowance, the level of intake of specific vitamins and minerals recommended each day to maintain good health. The values – and the terminology – vary slightly between different countries, for example the UK relies on DRVs (Dietary Reference Values), the EU has PRIs (Population Reference Intakes) and the US now uses DRIs (Dietary Reference Intakes) rather than RDAs.

Red blood cells Blood cells containing haemoglobin, which carry oxygen to and from body tissues and organs. Lack of red blood cells can cause fatigue and anaemia.

Resveratrol A flavonoid with both antioxidant and anti-inflammatory properties, found mainly in red wine.

Retinol Vitamin A.

Riboflavin Vitamin B2, one of the B vitamins involved in the body's production of energy.

Rutin A citrus flavonoid that works well with vitamin C. Found in buckwheat and many fruits.

Salicylates Naturally occurring aspirin-like compounds found in certain foods, for example almonds, strawberries and tomatoes.

Saponins Phytonutrients found in soya beans and soya products, which may lower LDL cholesterol and help protect against cancer.

Saturated fat A fat of animal origin (with the exception of palm oil, and coconut oil), which is solid at room temperature. Too much saturated fat in the diet raises blood cholesterol and increases the risk of heart disease.

Serotonin A neurotransmitter that helps regulate sleep patterns and mood. Low levels of serotonin are associated with depression.

Starchy foods Carbohydate foods with a high content of starch, for example bread, rice, pasta and potatoes.

Stroke A brain injury caused by disrupted blood supply to the brain via the cerebral arteries – in the same way that blocked arteries to the heart can cause heart attack.

Sulphoraphane A powerful compound found in brassicas that is effective in removing carcinogens from the body.

Superfoods Foods with alleged healing or health-promoting capabilities, also referred to as 'miracle foods'.

Synergy Two or more substances working in tandem to synergistic effect, whereby they achieve more in partnership than either could alone.

Tannin Antioxidant substance found in grape seeds, red wine and tea. Too much tannin reduces the body's ability to absorb iron.

Thiamin Vitamin B1, one of the B vitamins involved in the body's production of energy. Occurs in the outer coat of rice and other grains.

Tocopherol Vitamin E.

Toxins Harmful substances that may be consumed in food, or created by the body as a waste product and need to be eliminated.

Trans fats Very damaging type of fat produced during the hydrogenation process of turning unsaturated liquid fat (vegetable oils) into solid fat (margarine). High consumption of trans fats raises blood cholesterol and increases the risk of heart disease.

Tryptophan One of the essential amino acids. A component of proteins needed by the body for growth and a precursor of both serotonin and niacin.

Tyrosine See Amino acids.

Ultraviolet UV, an invisible band of radiation at the upper end of the visible light spectrum. Too much exposure to the sun's UV rays can damage the eyes, immune system and skin and can cause skin cancers, such as melanoma.

Unsaturated fat Group of fatty acids encompassing monounsaturated, polyunsaturated fats and the two essential fatty acids the body cannot make for itself, linoleic acid (omega-6) and alpha-linolenic acid (omega-3). Relatively healthy fats, which help reduce levels of blood cholesterol.

Uric acid A natural waste product derived from the breakdown of purines and usually eliminated from the body in the urine. Abnormal build-up of uric acid crystals in the body may result in gout, a painful condition in which certain joints become inflamed.

Vitamins Organic compounds required by the body in small quantities for normal health and development. There are two main types — fat-soluble vitamins (A, D, E and K), which are stored in the body, and water-soluble ones (vitamin C and the B complex vitamins). The latter are not stored in the body and so are required on a daily basis from food in the diet or via supplements.

White blood cells Large blood cells that are part of the immune system and help the body fight foreign invaders and infections.

Wholegrains Largely unprocessed nutrient-rich grain foods (for example whole or rolled oats, whole wheat, bulgur, or brown rice) that provide the maximum health benefits.

Zeaxanthin A type of carotenoid which, like lutein, promotes healthy eyes, reducing the risk of cataracts and age-related macular degeneration.

a

aduki beans 216
almonds 176–7
   garlic and almond soup
   222
amino acids 16, 25
anaemia 34
anchovies 194–5
animal proteins 16
anthocyanidins 24, 30
antioxidants 21, 23,
   24–5, 26
apples 40–1
   baked with lemon 40
   guava, apple and
   banana smoothie 65
apricots 60–1
artichokes, globe 148–9
asparagus 104–5
atherosclerosis 34
avocados 96–7
   endive and avocado
   salad 152
   mango, avocado and
   chicken salad 58

pink grapefruit and
   pine nut salad 48
salsa 96
smoked chicken and
   avocado salad 138

b

bacon, spinach and blue
   cheese salad 122
balanced diet 6, 11–13
bananas 44–5
   banana and peanut
   butter smoothie 44
   grilled fruit 55
   guava, apple and
   banana smoothie 65
   wheatgerm, pineapple
   and banana booster
   210
beans 216–17
   broad 110–11
   green 108–9
beef, green peppercorn
   steak 232
beetroot 142–3

betacarotene 20, 30
bhindi bhaji 114
biotin 30
blackberries 74–5
   blackberry and oat
   layer 74
   blueberry and
   blackberry yoghurt
   syllabub 164
blackcurrants 78–9
blood sugar levels 14–15,
   27, 29
blueberries 70–1
   and blackberry yoghurt
   syllabub 164
   porridge and nuts 178
   and raspberry brûlée
   70
Brazil nuts 170–1
bread 12
Breton crêpes 206
broad beans 110–11
broccoli 100–1
brown rice 204–5
Brussels sprouts 150–1

buckwheat 206–7
butternut squashes
   130–1

c

cabbage 132–3
calcium 22, 30
cancer 6, 24, 25, 26, 28,
   29, 32
cannellini bean and
   sundried tomato salad
   216
cantaloupe melons 90–1
carbohydrates 12, 14–15
carotenoids 24, 26
carrots 118–19
   carrot soup with
   orange and ginger 52
cashews 174–5
cauliflower 146–7
celeriac, spiced mackerel
   and celeriac mash
   188–9
cellulite 34
cereals 12

cheese 19, 28
  bacon, spinach and
    blue cheese salad
    122
  braised fennel with
    pecorino 120
  broad bean and
    pecorino salad 110
  fig, mozzarella and
    prosciutto salad 56
  fresh ricotta with herb
    oil and radishes 137
  pear and Stilton salad
    42
  watermelon and feta
    salad 88
cherries 82–3
chestnuts, Brussels
  sprouts with 151
chicken 27, 228–9
  cashew chicken 175
  mango, avocado and
    chicken salad 58
  with rosemary and
    garlic 228
  smoked chicken and
    avocado salad 138
chickpeas 212–13
  chickpea cakes 170
chicory 152–3
chillies 218–19
Chinese cabbage, stir
  fried 133

chocolate 29
cholesterol 18, 27, 36
chromium 22, 23, 30
chutney, fresh chilli 218
clafoutis, cherry 82
colcannon 141
colds 34
constipation 27, 35
cooking, healthy
  32
copper (trace mineral)
  23, 30
cranberries 80–1
cucumber seaweed and
  cucumber salad 103
  strawberry and
    cucumber salad 76

d
dairy products 12, 13,
  16
dates 86–7
depression 35
dhal 215
diverticulosis 27
dried apricots 60

e
Earl Grey brûlée
  238
eggs 28, 166–7
  boiled eggs with
    anchovy soldiers 195

watercress and
  mushroom frittata
  167
endive 152–3
essential fatty acids 18,
  27, 30
exhaustion 35

f
fatigue 35
fats 12, 13, 18–19
fennel 120–1
fertility 36
fibre 15, 27
figs 56–7
  fig and molasses cake
    bars 157
fish and shellfish 13,
  27–8, 188–203
flavonoids 24, 26
flaxseed 186–7
fluoride 23, 30
folate (folic acid) 21,
  30
food pyramid 12
free radicals 24, 25
fresh herbs 224–5
fruit 12, 25, 26, 26–7,
  40–91
  cooking 32
  grilled 55
  hot fruit salad
    84

g
game fowl 230–1
garlic 222–3
  chicken with rosemary
    and 228
GI (glycaemic index) 15
ginger 220–1
  carrot soup with
    orange and 52
  mangetout with ginger
    and mint 112
globe artichokes 148–9
glucosinolates 24
glycaemic index (GI) 15
gout 35
grains 28–9, 210–11
grapefruit 48–9
  black grape jelly with
    citrus fruits 47
  and prawn salad 172
grapes 46–7
grazing 13
green beans 108–9
green peppercorn steak
  232
green tea 238
guavas 64–5
guinea fowl, grilled
  230

h
hangovers 35
hazelnuts 172–3

HDL (highdensity lipoprotein) 18
healthy eating 10–14
heart disease 6, 18, 19, 28
herbs, fresh 224–5
high blood pressure (hypertension) 35–6
honey 28, 154–5
 honeyed granola 184
 and yoghurt with prune purée 154
horseradish 226–7

i
ice cream, quinoa coconut 209
immune system 25
insomnia 36
iodine (trace mineral) 23, 30
iron 22, 23, 30
irritable bowel syndrome (IBS) 36
isoflavones 30

j
jelly, black grape jelly with citrus fruits 47

k
kale 140–1
Kerala prawn curry 196
kiwi fruit 62–3

l
LDL (lowdensity lipoprotein) 18
lean red meat 232–3
lemons 50–1
 apples baked with lemon 40
 lemon and basil penne 51
lentils 214–15
lettuce 138–9
lignans 23, 25, 29, 30
limes 50–1
linseed (flaxseed) 186–7
live yoghurt 29, 164–5
liver 236–7
lycopene 30

m
mackerel 188–9
magnesium 22, 23, 30
manganese 23, 25, 30
mangetout 112–13
mangoes 58–9
 grilled fruit 55
 mango, avocado and chicken salad 58

meat 13, 27, 28, 232–3
Mediterranean diet 6
melons
 cantaloupe melons 90–1
 kiwi fruit, melon and grape salad 63
 watermelons 88–9
menopausal problems 36–7
milk 16, 22, 29, 162–3
 junket with rhubarb 162
minerals 21, 22–3
molasses 28, 156–7
monounsaturated fats 19
muffins, cranberry 80
mung beans 216
mushrooms 124–5
 watercress and mushroom frittata 167
mussels 200–1

n
nutrients 10, 14–23, 30–1
 preserving 32–3
nuts 29, 168–77

o
oats 178–9
 apricots poached with oatmeal cream 60

blackberry and oat layer 74
 sweet oat cakes 159
oily fish 27–8
okra 114–15
olive oil 28, 158–9
olives 158–9
omega 3 essential fatty acids 27, 30
omega 6 essential fatty acids 30
onions 98–9
oranges 52–3
 black grape jelly with citrus fruits 47
 carrot soup with orange and ginger 52
 date and orange fool 86
 grilled fruit 55
organic food 33
osteoarthritis 37
osteoporosis 37
Oxygen Radical Absorbance Capacity (ORAC) 25
oysters 198–9

p
papayas 54–5
partridge 230

passionfruit, raspberry and passionfruit fool 72

pasta 12
  beetroot and sugar snap 142
  lemon and basil penne 51

peach and tofu smoothie 161

pears 42–3
  chilled watercress and pear soup 134

peas 106–7

peppers 116–17

pheasant 230

phosphorus 22, 23, 31

phytonutrients 10, 24–5, 30–1

pine nuts, pink grapefruit and pine nut salad 48

pineapples 66–7
  baked pineapple rings with cinnamon 67
  wheatgerm, pineapple and banana booster 210

plums 84–5

polyunsaturated fats 19

pomegranates 68–9

potassium 23, 31

potatoes 12, 144–5
  colcannon 141
  horseradish mash 227

prawns 196–7
  grapefruit and prawn salad 172

premenstrual syndrome (PMS) 37

pregnant women 21, 27–8

processed food 32

prostate gland problems 37

protein foods 12, 13, 16–17

prunes 84–5
  honey and yoghurt with prune purée 154

pulses 28–9, 212–17

pumpkin seeds 182–3

pumpkins 130–1

q

Quark 19

quinoa 208–9

r

radishes 136–7

raspberries 72–3
  blueberry and raspberry brûlée 70
  melon with 91
  and passionfruit fool 72

rheumatoid arthritis 37

rhubarb, milk junket with 162

rice
  brown 204–5
  herby risotto 224
  spring onion and ginger 220

s

salads
  bacon, spinach and blue cheese 122
  broad bean and pecorino 110
  endive and avocado 152
  fig, mozzarella and prosciutto 56
  grapefruit and prawn 172
  green bean and tomato 108
  hot fruit 84
  kiwi fruit, melon and grape 63
  mango, avocado and chicken 58
  pear and Stilton 42
  pink grapefruit and pine nut 48
  pomegranate and mixed leaf 68

seared scallops with lime dressed 202

seaweed and cucumber 103

smoked chicken and avocado 138

spiced chickpea 212

watermelon and feta 88

salmon 192–3

salsa
  avocado 96
  baked sweet potatoes with 128
  tomato and coriander 93

sardines 188–9

saturated fats 18

scallops 202–3

seasonal produce 33

seaweed 102–3

seeds 29, 180–7, 206–9

selenium 23, 25, 29, 31

sesame seeds 184–5

shopping for food 33

silicon 31

sodium 23, 31

soups
  artichoke and dill 148
  carrot soup with orange and ginger 52
  chilled watercress and pear 134

garlic and almond 222
smooth onion 98
summer green pea 107
soya 160–1
soya beans 216
spinach 122–3
spirulina 29
spring onion and ginger rice 220
squashes 130–1
starchy foods 14–15
storing food 33
strawberries 76–7
and cucumber salad 76
stress 37
sugars 12, 13, 14–15
sulforaphane 31
sunflower seeds 180–1
walnut and sunflower seed stacks 168

sweet potatoes 128–9
sweetcorn 94–5

t
tea 28, 238–9
tofu 28, 160–1
tomatoes 92–3
green bean and tomato salad 108
trans fats 18
tryptophan 36
tuna 190–1
turkey 228–9

v
vegetable proteins 16
vegetables 12, 25–6, 94–153
cooking 32
venison 234–5

Vitamin A 20, 25, 31
Vitamin B complex 20–1, 25, 31
Vitamin C 10, 21, 25, 31
and iron 23
Vitamin D 20, 31
Vitamin E 10, 20, 25, 29, 31
Vitamin K 20, 31
vitamin supplements 21
vitamins 10, 18, 19, 20–1

w
walnuts 168–9
roasted pumpkin with walnut and rocket pesto 130

walnut and sunflower seed stacks 168
watercress 134–5
and mushroom frittata 167
watermelons 88–9
wheatgerm 210–11

y
yams 126–7
yoghurt 29, 164–5

z
zinc 22, 23, 25, 31

acknowledgements

Executive Editor Nicola Hill
Editor Lisa John
Design Manager Tokiko Morishima
Designer Jo MacGregor
Home Economist Mary Wall
Senior Production Controller Manjit Sihra

Special Photography © **Octopus Publishing Group Limited**/Stephen Conroy.
Other Photography © **Octopus Publishing Group Limited**/Jeremy Hopley 165, 223, 231; William Lingwood 106, 180, 197, 205.